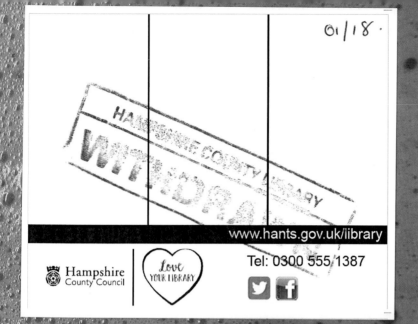

TONIC

Tanita de Ruijt

TONIC

DELICIOUS & NATURAL REMEDIES
TO BOOST YOUR HEALTH

Photography By Patricia Niven

hardie grant books

Contents

INTRODUCTION

Every year, at the first sign of a stuffy nose, I head to my kitchen for help. I'll mix up one of my signature tonics to quickly put me right. No, I'm not a doctor, or a nutritionist for that matter; nor do I plan on becoming either. I'm just a home cook – one who is fully invested in unlocking both the flavour and the medicinal potential of my ingredients.

Using food as medicine is part of a basic instinct for survival that we seem to have lost touch with. It's a handy one, too, especially when life throws you one of its many curveballs, such as waking up with a sore throat on the day of an important meeting; overeating and feeling bloated (life's too delicious); waking up with a hangover (it happens); or the classic afternoon slump.

There was a time when all cooks were also experts on medicinal foods. Herbs and spices served a dual purpose – they went into medicinal concoctions as well as into the cooking pot; into the types of homemade remedies your grandma used to make. I call them tonics.

Incorporating tonics into your lifestyle could help to prevent symptoms by supporting your body's basic systems such as the digestive, respiratory, nervous, and endocrine system. Tonics support these systems by tackling everyday ailments before they become visible or start to develop into something more significant. It is a preventative and all-encompassing approach to health.

Importantly, making a tonic is not about having all the latest healthy 'superfoods' on hand. A lot of the most potent ingredients, such as herbs and spices, already sit in our kitchen cupboards. Their smells alone can entice the appetite, activate digestion, and release feel-good endorphins.

This book offers all-natural, diverse ways to treat basic ailments quickly, safely, and effectively at home. These tonics will tickle your taste buds, raise your energy, and elevate your mood.

Discover ways to pillage your kitchen cupboards and make surprisingly effective – and inexpensive – remedies.

THE JAMU KITCHEN

Although I grew up in the south of Spain, my real culinary journey didn't actually begin until a visit to Bali, Indonesia, where I took a walk around an organic farm. It was the way the unassuming guide, probably in his mid-50s, talked about his ingredients, that changed my approach to health completely.

He picked a fresh bay leaf from a tree and told me how he planned to brew it up later to make evening tea, to help relieve his aching joints after the long day spent harvesting on the farm. I had been expecting him to talk about how it would make a great addition to a rendang curry – we were foraging for our lunch after all. For him, it wasn't all about flavour. This humble knowledge about the medicinal potential of an ingredient was considered vital information, passed down from generation to generation. He called it 'Jamu'. I found it fascinating.

Jamu is the traditional system of medicine in Indonesia. It relies on the use of local roots, spices, herbs, barks, plants and peels to support our general wellbeing. It was relied upon before the arrival of Western medicine, and was greatly influenced by the basic principles of Chinese medicine and Ayurveda, yet adapted to suit the varied tropical plants of the incredibly bio-diverse archipelago that is Indonesia.

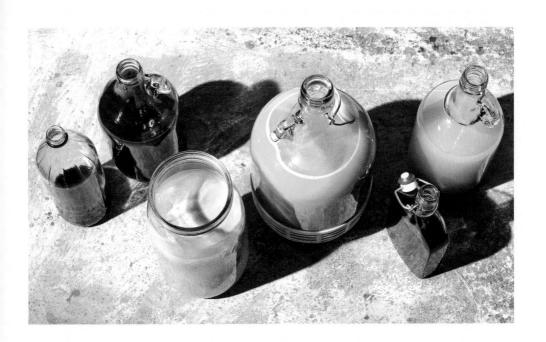

*Turmeric tamarind tonic
(Jamu Kunyit Asam)
is the most popular
remedy within this
system. It is said to
purify the blood, support
liver detoxification,
reduce inflammation,
fight off bacteria,
improve immunity
and aid in slimming.*

Despite its power, it is a modest tonic, sold hawker-style on the streets to neighbours and friends. I drank it every morning during my stay and, eventually, one of the vendors agreed to show me how she makes hers.

After returning to London, I began making *Jamu* at home, with the most similar ingredients that I could find. Next thing I knew, I was selling a few bottles at a market in South London on the weekends for fun. That's how I started the 'Jamu Kitchen'.

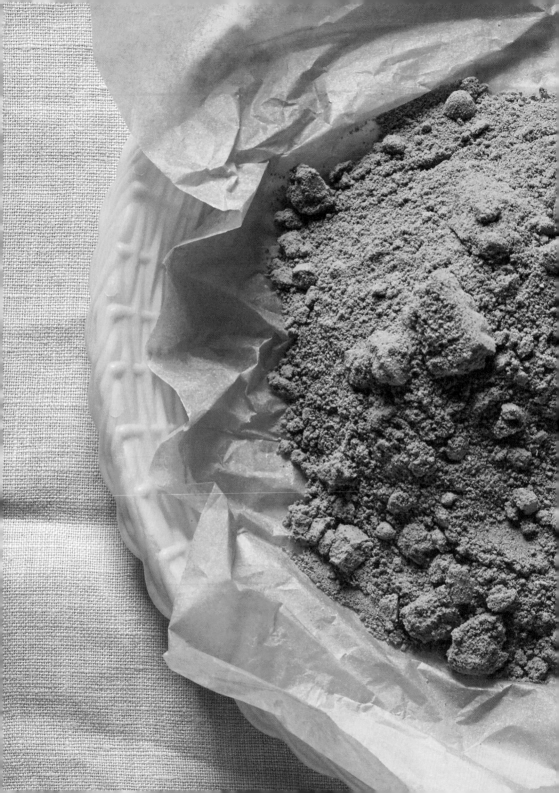

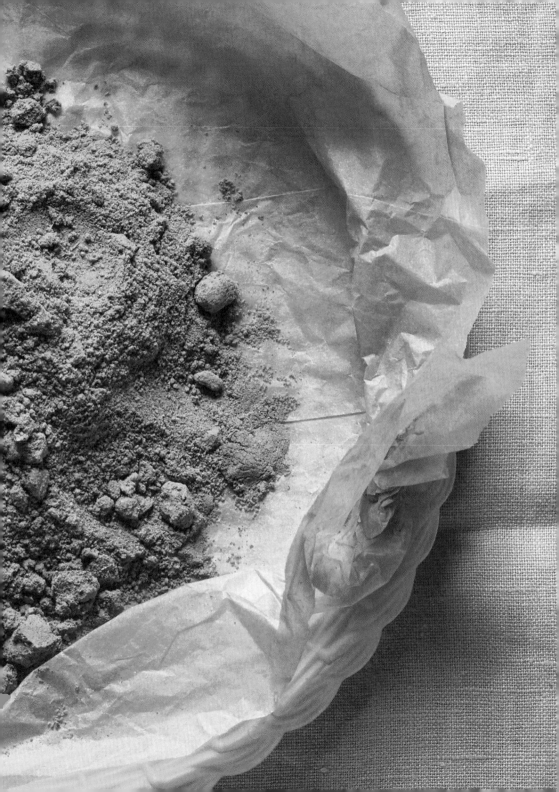

ANCIENT WISDOM — MODERN TIMES

The burning ambition behind Jamu Kitchen is the idea that, in one way or another, I am doing my part to preserve an incredibly valuable traditional food culture, and simultaneously increasing awareness of it, by making the concept of drinking medicinal tonic more accessible. Seeing a drink that I found on the back streets of Bali on a shop shelf in London was a small step towards that goal.

Now, I am writing this book to pay the information I have accumulated forward; to help others understand the potential of humble ingredients; to enable them to feel confident in starting their own *Jamu* kitchen; and ultimately to help them become better equipped when it comes to self-care.

Science is only starting to catch up with what our ancestors have known for centuries. My tonic recipes are guided by new breakthroughs in the West, as well as by old food wisdoms in their purest state, primarily from the East. Some have legitimate science going for them – all have a strong, folk-medicine track record.

Although I place a lot of emphasis on the importance of preserving tradition, my eclectic list of recipes has been adapted to suit the needs and tastes of today, without compromising any medicinal potential. Flavour plays a key part in this evolution, as eating and drinking things we enjoy is, naturally, a much more sustainable way to incorporate them into our lifestyles. (A good example of this is the way 'gin and tonic' was born: British army officers serving in India found that the bitter quinine in the tonic water they consumed to avoid malaria could be made more palatable if they added gin and lime to the mix.)

ABOUT THIS BOOK

I encourage you to experiment with the recipes to adapt them to your tastes or lifestyle. There are no rules (apart from those in the next few paragraphs). Find out what works for you.

This book is divided into two parts. The first part is a guide to the medicinal potential of the roots, barks, peels, herbs and spices needed to make a tonic. It tells you everything you need to start your very own experimental apothecary kitchen.

The second part is an array of recipes that will demonstrate how to pack these ingredients into your life, effortlessly, when they're needed the most. Some are quick and easy to make, others will take time and patience to get right. The chapters are divided into the way you're feeling, to help you pick what's right for you.

These recipes are intended for basic self-care, in order keep you feeling good on a daily basis. If you are ill beyond the ailments outlined in this book, I suggest you visit a doctor.

PRINCIPLES

When we separate pleasure from nutrition in our diets, we end up less nourished both physically and emotionally. Enjoying what you eat and drink is good for you.

Flavour can also heal. Each taste has a therapeutic effect on the body. Tonics are a great and easy way to incorporate all of these tastes into your lifestyle on a regular basis.

Bitterness The key quality of a tonic. Tonics are bitter by nature, and it's this taste that stimulates all of our bodily systems (see also p. 110)

QUALITY

A tonic can only be as good as its ingredients – only settle for the best. If you're leaving skins on roots, or using the fresh herbs, you must make sure they are pesticide-free. Whole spices are best bought whole, so their potent oils are kept intact. If you drink milk, it's best drunk whole and non-homogenised, from happy cows. Sugars and salts should be natural, unrefined and used in moderation. Make the most of your waste. Hold on to your peels, rinds and barks – they will come in handy too.

Sweetness Sugar helps strengthen, moisten and harmonise many systems of our body, especially when we are at our weakest. It also helps to make tonics more palatable. Be good to yourself.

Saltiness Salt is essential for sustaining hydration and maintaining a good balance of electrolytes to keep our organs functioning smoothly. These electrolytes include magnesium, potassium, calcium, and sodium.

Sourness The acidity of sour ingredients triggers the digestive process, activating the salivary glands, stimulating the appetite, and improving the absorption of the essential nutrients in what you are eating or drinking.

BALANCE

All good things are better in moderation. Even a good thing can become destructive if taken to excess. Try to incorporate these ingredients and tonics when it seems right, or tasty – that way it becomes a much more organic, varied, flavoursome and sustainable process that's been led primarily by your intuition and the way that you feel.

Spiciness helps to increase your body heat, invigorate the blood, boost the metabolism, and encourage weight loss, as well as suppress aches and pains. It is perfect for treating common colds.

INSIDE THE JAMU APOTHECARY KITCHEN

*This is a short
guide to the simplest
kitchen gifts that
keep on giving
– a breakdown of the
essential ingredients
and tools that you will
need to start your
own apothecary kitchen.*

Given the humble nature and wide availability of a lot of these ingredients, most of us wouldn't automatically recognise them as medicinal, let alone know which parts to use or what to do with them.

Herbs and spices all originate from plants: flowers, fruits, seeds, barks, leaves and roots. They have anti-inflammatory, antibacterial and antiviral properties and contain more disease-fighting antioxidants than most fruits and vegetables. Antioxidants are the body's defence agents. They are chemical compounds that prevent ageing and chronic diseases. Put simply, the more you have, the better equipped your body will be to fight off infections and diseases.

TOOLS

PESTLE AND MORTAR
I have a thing for the pestle and mortar.
It's not just decorative – it's the ultimate
kitchen tool: perfect for smashing up ginger
or lemongrass; for grinding whole spices
into powders; for bruising herbs, and so
much more.

The pestle and mortar was the first tool
used to make medicine, and is still used
today. The first record of one dates to
1550 BC in the Ebers Papyrus. The Egyptians
and Persians both used them for culinary
and medicinal purposes. It became the
symbol of the ancient apothecary and the
modern pharmacist.

BLENDER
The modern version of a pestle and mortar
will also come in handy. Just because the
ancients didn't have a food processor,
doesn't mean you can't use one! Get a
high-powered blender and an additional
blender cup for your turmeric concoctions
(it will stain).

**SWING-TOP
(STOPPERED) BOTTLES**
For storing your tonics. These keep the
valuable CO_2 gases produced by fermentation (the bubbles) firmly sealed within the
bottle. See also the note about sterilisation
(right).

MEASURING JUGS (PITCHERS)
Glass is best – plastics will stain.

SCALES
Digital preferably, although not essential.

**LARGE MASON (SCREW-TOP
PRESERVING) JARS**
For steeping and brewing the fizzy fermented tonics. Kilner do
great ones.

MUSLIN (CHEESECLOTH)
For filtering and fermenting.

ELASTIC BANDS
For sealing.

FINE-MESH SIEVE (STRAINER)
For filtering.

STAINLESS-STEEL PANS
Because turmeric will stain anything else.

PLASTIC OR SILICONE GLOVES
Same reason as above.

INTUITION

All things fermented and somewhat funky require some initiative. There are wild yeasts involved that co-exist with plenty of other micro-organisms, including a substantial amount of acetic acid bacteria. These are essential for developing refreshingly funky tonics, but there can be other, less welcome, bacteria that can develop in your batch, too. If your batch smells foul or starts to grow mould, get rid of it, and start over.

TIME

Tonic-making isn't always quick. It's about adding more, never taking anything out; making upgrades, not sacrifices.

STERILISATION

Sterilise the bottles you plan to store your tonics in. It prevents any nasty bacteria from interfering with them.

1. Clean bottles in a white vinegar solution. Fill a large bowl with half hot water and half white vinegar. Let your bottles soak in this solution for 20 minutes. While they are soaking, give each a good scrub with a bottle brush.

2. After soaking and washing, boil your bottles for 10 minutes in a large saucepan (making sure the bottles are completely submerged and there are no trapped air bubbles). This is a secondary measure to ensure that the bottle is completely clean. It also removes any excess vinegar from the surface of the bottles.

3. Dry your bottles well before use by placing in a low oven.

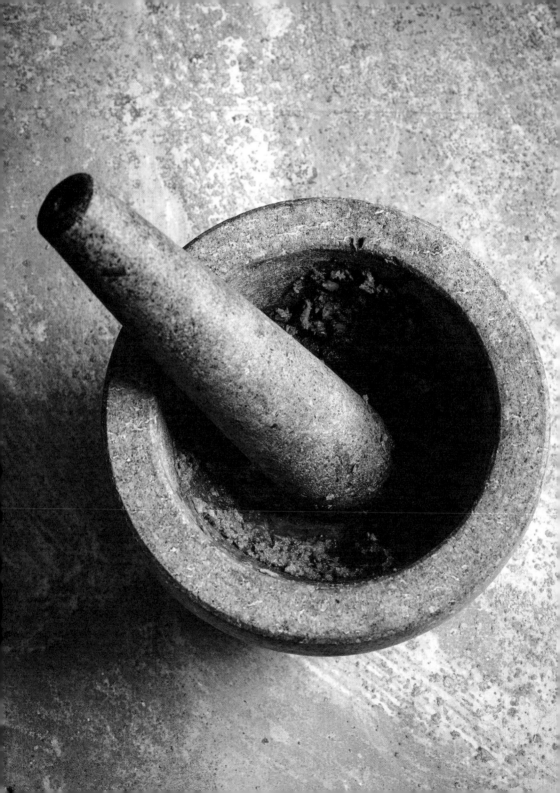

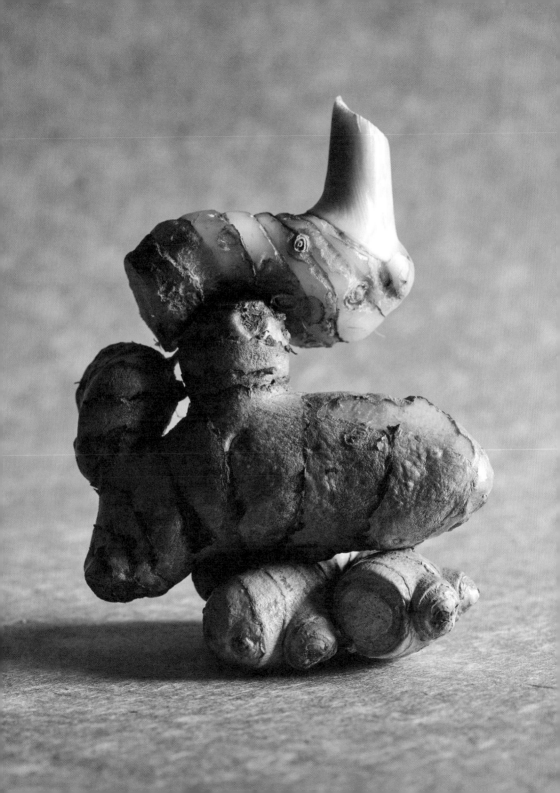

THE 3 GINGERS

Ginger is the undisputed hero of the apothecary kitchen. The name actually applies to a whole family of roots, that come in a variety of shapes and colours, with different flavours and benefits.

Turmeric and galangal are both a type of ginger. They are among the most popular ingredients used for medicinal purposes around the world.

A remarkable number of different tonics are made using various combinations of basic gingers. The roots will be ground into a fine paste and other medicinal herbs and spices will be added for their cumulative effects. Each combination creates a unique tonic to cure different ailments.

TURMERIC

Turmeric is king when it comes to spice. Its yellow colour has long been considered sacred in the Eastern world. Yellow symbolises the sun – a source of light, energy and growth – which is why this colour is associated with royalty and is believed to offer protection from evil spirits throughout Asia.

Benefits This lively root is highly praised for its healing powers. It has antibacterial, antifungal and antiviral properties, due to an active chemical called curcumin, which can reduce inflammation. Regular consumption of turmeric helps to protect the digestive system, cleanse the blood and improve circulation. Turmeric is found in almost every traditional *Jamu* recipe.

Fresh turmeric The roots look similar to ginger and, like ginger, fresh roots have a zingier flavour than dried. Turmeric's bright orange flesh tastes earthy, citrusy, peppery and slightly bitter.

Ground turmeric The ground variety is made by peeling, boiling, drying and grinding the roots. It loses some of its essential oils and pungency during these processes but it will still provide a lot of warmth and colour for meals.

Fresh vs. Dried For the best flavour and medicinal qualities, stick to fresh. A great way to store fresh turmeric (and fresh ginger or galangal) is in the freezer. Pull out a piece when you need one. It only needs to thaw for a few minutes before it is ready to slice.

As a general rule: 2.5 cm (1 in) fresh turmeric root = 1 tablespoon freshly grated turmeric = 1 teaspoon ground turmeric

Preparation Rinse roots thoroughly, leaving the skin on, as there's plenty of good stuff in there too. Grind into a paste, as needed, using a microplane grater, pestle and mortar, or blender. Grinding is the key to maximising surface area and getting the most nutritional potential out of your roots.

Be warned – fresh turmeric stains easily, so unless you want to turn your kitchen yellow, handle with care. Wear gloves and avoid using plastics. In that event, all is not lost: lemon juice helps to remove turmeric stains from your hands.

How to consume turmeric Roots and spices are all about synergy – pairing them creates more than just great flavour, it also makes them a lot more bioavailable. Pairing turmeric with other complementary flavours, with spices such as ginger and black pepper, or fats such as coconut oil or milk, has been scientifically proven to increase our body's ability to absorb the benefits of turmeric. Brewing, or warming, your turmeric also makes it easier to digest and more bioavailable too.

GINGER

The best-known member of the family: primarily for its flavour, but also for protecting and promoting a healthy digestive system. It's one of the oldest medicinal plants used in Chinese, Ayurvedic and Indonesian medicine. According to these systems, ginger warms the body, eases nausea, revs up the appetite and digestion, helps ward off any aches and pains, and restores strength to those suffering from illness. Steeped hot ginger teas help relieve symptoms of cold and flu. When combined with turmeric, its effects multiply. The skin can be left on, as long as it is rinsed properly.

GALANGAL

The lesser-known member of the pack, galangal root is more aromatic than its cousin ginger. Galangal's origins can be traced back to Hainan in China, where it has been used for thousands of years in Chinese medicine. It shares several healing properties with ginger, such as warming the body, aiding digestion and preventing nausea.

In the 19th century, St. Hildegard, a renowned healer and expert in herbal medicine, recognised galangal's healing qualities and dubbed it the 'spice of life'. He considered it to be a cure-all for many of the diseases that ravaged Europe during this time.

Although fresh galangal is harder to find, it's definitely worth the trouble. All of these roots can be found in Asian supermarkets.

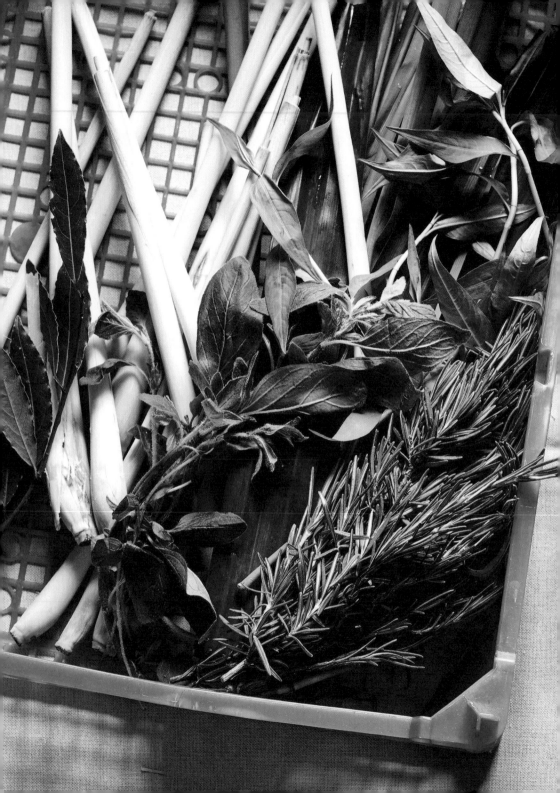

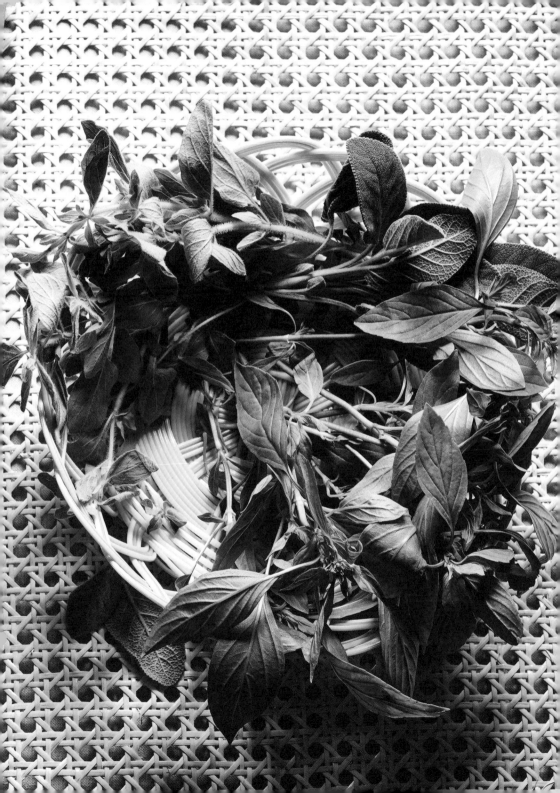

HERBS

Take a pick-and-mix approach to your herbs, depending on your discomforts, or what you have lying around from your previous night's meal, to make an invigorating tonic to cure your ailments.

Spanking fresh, leafy herbs is a necessary discipline. Don't crush them into a paste – just give them a quick, firm slap. Overly bruising herbs makes them taste bitter and grassy, so go easy. Strike them just hard enough to activate all those aromatic essential oils. Then, steep them in hot water to make the ultimate fresh herbal tea tonic. You'll never look back at the dried stuff.

LEMONGRASS

An aromatic healer with a distinct lemony flavour and citrusy aroma, lemongrass is nature's paracetamol: it reduces pain and inflammation; it helps to bring down high fevers; and relieves headaches. It's known as 'fevergrass' in Jamaica. Lemongrass also helps to restore our vital systems, including digestion, respiration, excretion and the nervous system.

Helps with: detoxification, reducing cholesterol, digestion, stress, fevers, headaches and pains, infections and immune system

BASIL

Italian basil, Thai basil, holy basil; it's all basil baby. Each type is incredibly healthy and packed with strong antioxidant and antimicrobial activity, yet it varies in flavour. It is traditionally thought to stimulate the appetite and ease stomach discomfort, soothing indigestion and alleviating feelings of fullness. It also helps to alleviate symptoms of stress and tense headaches.

Holy basil, in particular, has endless miraculous and medicinal values that have been worshiped and highly valued across India for thousands of years. If you can find it fresh, you're in luck.

Helps with: brain function and memory, digestive discomfort and stress

MINT

There are over fifteen varieties of magnificent medicinal mints, from peppermint and spearmint to pineapple mint – all equally healthy. Mint is cooling and calming, and traditionally used to treat digestive discomfort, as well as colds, flu and stuffy noses, thanks to its ability to open the sinuses and, in combination with honey, to ease sore throats.

Helps with: digestion, nausea and headaches, congestion, depression, fatigue and weight loss

THYME

Highly valued for relieving coughs, colds and congestion, thyme is very rich in essential oils that have the ability to prevent fungal and viral infections, therefore reducing pressure on the immune system. Thyme is also packed with vitamin C – so, if you feel a cold coming on, this herb will help put you right in no thyme.

Helps with: coughs and sore throats, congestion, immune system and stress

SAGE

The name comes from the Latin word *salvere*, meaning 'to be saved'. Sage leaves are used to make medicines which improve digestion, memory and symptoms of depression. They're packed with essential oils that enhance mental clarity and improve the memory. Steep them in hot water for a 'thinker's tea'.

Helps with: stomach pain, memory loss, stress and bloating

OREGANO

The name means 'mountain joy', and oregano was revered as a symbol of happiness by the ancient Greeks and Romans. In the 19th century, herbal doctors prescribed oregano as a general well-being tonic to promote menstruation. It's also used to treat respiratory issues, such as stuffy noses and coughs, and digestive issues.

Helps with: digestive issues, bacterial infections, menstruation and colds and flu

BAY

Bay leaves contain a very strong diuretic that stimulates urination, in order to decrease the toxicity of the body. They are also very effective for settling upset stomachs, and soothing painful joints.

Helps with: detoxifying, ageing, inflammation in joints, digestion and anxiety and stress

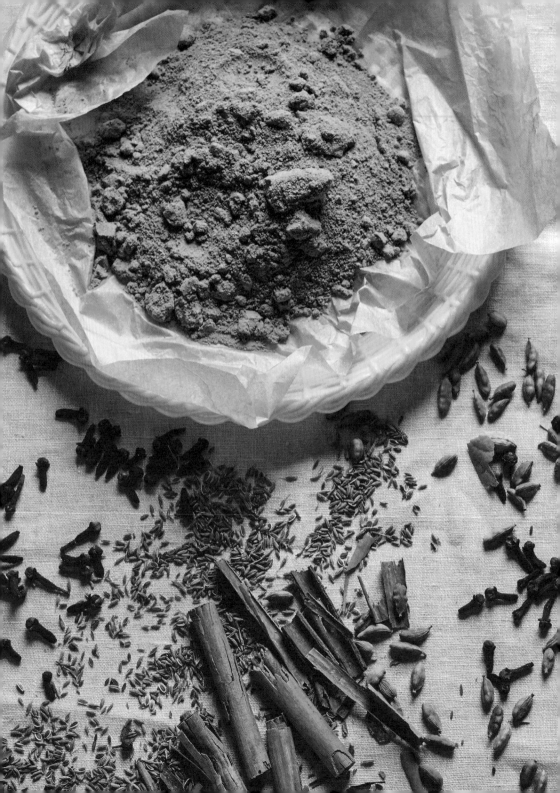

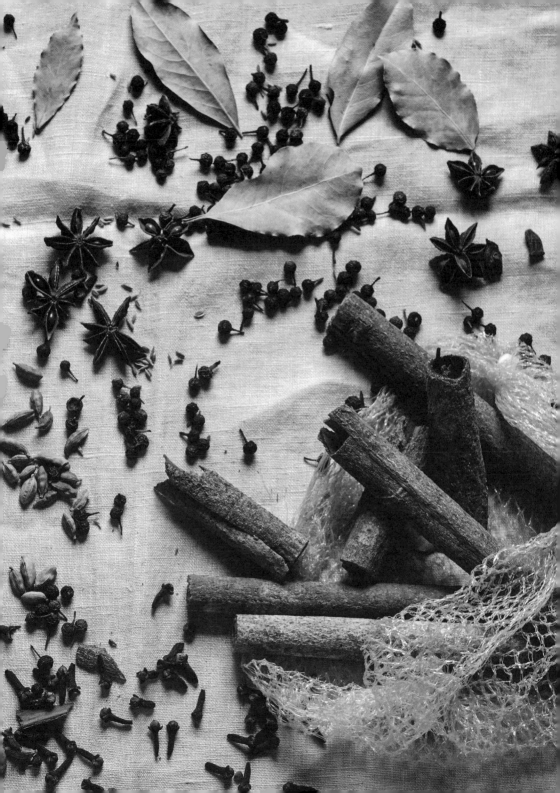

SPICES

Welcome to the spice rack, a.k.a. your new medicine cabinet, brimming with flavour-packed remedies.

Whole spices are preferred, but ground will do just fine. Ground spices are less potent, as they tend to lose their essential oils over time. Spices should be treated the same way we treat coffee beans.

1. Heat - If using whole spices, dry-fry or toast them in a pan, until they become aromatic – this will activate their medicinal oils and properties.

2. Grind - Grinding spices will lower the amount of time needed to steep them, and help them release their essential oils more readily.

3. Add fats - The elements that make spices taste delicious are all aromatic compounds. You'll need full fat (whole) milks and oils in order to extract as many flavours and benefits from them as you can. So, do your spices a favour and don't concoct a tonic with skimmed milk – try adding a dollop of coconut oil to your herbal brews.

Sidenote - The pungency of your spice is a good indicator of how much to use. Spices such as clove and nutmeg are very pungent, and should be used in moderation.

BLACK PEPPER

According to Ayurveda, the pungency and heat of black pepper work to help metabolise food as it is digested in our system. Its warming qualities also help to clear congestion in the respiratory system. Use for indigestion, sinus congestion, excess toxin build-up, fever, sluggish metabolism and obesity.

Helps with: digestion, congestion, cold and flu and weight loss

CINNAMON

An antibacterial spice found in most households, cinnamon increases general vitality, warms the body, counteracts congestion, improves digestion, relieves menstrual cramping and improves circulation. Look for Sri Lankan 'Ceylon cinnamon' *(cinnamomum verum)*, also known as 'true cinnamon', not cassia bark (Chinese cinnamon, *cinnamomum cassia*). Grate the bark straight into your concoctions.

Helps with: circulation, digestion, bacterial infections and menstruation

CLOVE

Cloves are the aromatic flower buds of a medicinal tree once indigenous to the Indonesian 'spice islands'. Also found in the spice racks of most homes, cloves are known to have antiseptic, anaesthetic, anti-inflammatory, warming, soothing and flatulence-relieving properties.

Helps with: indigestion, gas and bloating

CARDAMOM

Known as 'the queen of spices', cardamom is related to ginger. Like ginger, it's good for improving digestion, soothing stomach pains and relieving gas. Its warming properties also help to cleanse the body, and improve circulation. You will have to break open the pods to discover its plethora of health benefits.

Helps with: digestion, cholesterol, depression and inflammation

FENNEL SEED

Ancient cultures revered fennel, for its liquorice aroma and sweet taste, as well as its healing properties. Fennel seed is highly regarded for its ability to ease uncomfortable feelings of fullness, bloating or gassiness, and as an all-round promoter of healthy digestion. Chew these seeds to freshen the breath post-meal.

Helps with: digestion, bloating and overindulgence

CORIANDER SEED

A pleasant, aromatic and spicy seed with flatulence-relieving properties, it has been traditionally used to reduce gas in the stomach and intestines, and to stimulate digestion. In both traditional Chinese medicine and Ayurvedic medicine, coriander seeds are often combined with cardamom and fennel to treat digestive complaints.

Helps with: digestion and bloating

CUMIN

The cumin seed was once thought to promote love and fidelity – it was thrown around at weddings, and soldiers were even sent off to battle with a fresh loaf of cumin-seed bread. It's traditionally used as a carminative, to help settle the stomach, and ease bloating and trapped wind.

Helps with: bloating and flatulence

STAR ANISE

Used in traditional Chinese medicine to fight flu by clearing mucous from the respiratory tract, this spice is effective in fighting viral, bacterial or fungal infections, as well as inflammation. It's also a common ingredient in medicinal teas, to treat coughs and chest infections. The seeds can be chewed before meals to stimulate the appetite, or afterwards to relieve gas and bloating.

Helps with: inflammation and cold and flu

NUTMEG

Nutmeg acts as a tonic in many different ways, from its ability to relieve pain, soothe indigestion, strengthen cognitive function, detoxify the body, boost skin health, alleviate oral conditions, reduce anxiety and insomnia, and strengthen the immune system.

Helps with: stress and anxiety, mental health, digestion and aches

STAPLES

APPLE CIDER VINEGAR
Vinegar made from crushed apples fermented in wooden barrels, this is an alkalising agent that helps to balance your body's pH. Look for raw ACP, 'with the mother' – this means it hasn't been pasteurised and is still packed with beneficial acetic acid, potassium, magnesium, probiotics and enzymes. The 'mother' is the culture of beneficial bacteria that turns apple cider into vinegar in the first place. It's similar to the SCOBY (which is also called a 'mother') needed to make kombucha (see p. 118).

APPLE CIDER VINEGAR BITTERS
To give any drink an immediate bitter tonic quality (see p. 110).

CACAO
Cacao is the product of raw, fermented cacao beans – nothing else. Powdered or nibbed, it's said to impart a surge of brain-boosting endorphins, tons of energy, and a flood of magnesium that relaxes the body. This 'drug' can be ingested, drunk and even snorted. Cacao was apparently used by ancient cultures such as the Mayans to elevate their senses so they could commune with their God.

CHILLIES – FRESH OR DRIED
The heat you feel from cayenne pepper and chilli powder comes from capsaicin, a compound that has been shown to invigorate the blood, clear the nasal passages, and thin mucus. Fresh chillies also pack more vitamin C than oranges.

COCONUT OIL
Referred to as the 'tree of life' among tropical cultures, virtually all parts of the coconut palm have found use in traditional foods and medicines. Its oil, milk, cream and water is used for its antifungal, antibacterial and antiviral properties, which also help in dealing with various bacteria, fungi, and parasites that cause indigestion, and help to strengthen the immune system. Its fatty compounds make nutrients more bioavailable, increase the metabolism, and help with weight loss. Quality is key – look for unrefined, virgin coconut oil.

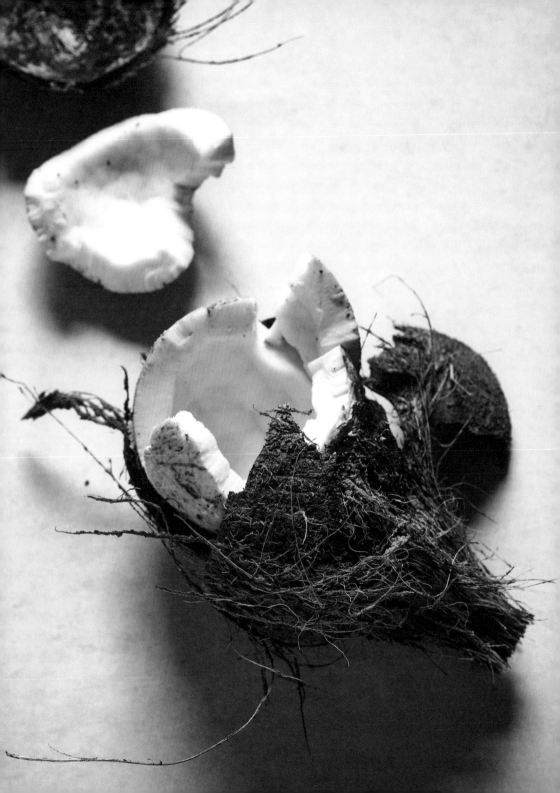

FERMENTED HONEY

Honey, made even better (see p. 144). Fermented honey harbours healthy yeasts and bacteria, and can therefore be used as a digestive aid and immunity booster.

GARLIC

Aphrodisiac, currency, food, medicine, vampire repellent – garlic has had many uses in many cultures for thousands of years. Its pungent sulphurs and antibacterial and anti-inflammatory properties are used to prevent colds and flu and treat a wide range of conditions and diseases.

GHEE (CLARIFIED BUTTER)

Use this clarified butter for a better gut. Ghee is a staple anti-inflammatory in Ayurvedic medicine, it is used to heal the digestive system. It is a traditionally held belief that, the older the ghee, the better its healing qualities. Aged ghee is often kept in temples in large vats and families often pass on aged ghee to the next generation to be used as medicine.

ONIONS

Onions have been used to reduce inflammation and heal infections for centuries. They're also one of the healthiest foods you can eat. A natural antihistamine, onions are also rich in vitamin C, sulphuric compounds, flavonoids, and other phytochemicals that can soothe the throat and clear stuffed-up nasal passages. An onion a day may help keep the doctor away.

SCOBY

Symbiotic Culture of Bacteria and Yeast – this is needed to transform sweet tea into tangy, fizzy kombucha (see p. 118).

TAMARIND

Deliciously tangy, tamarind is traditionally used to help stomach and digestive ailments, fevers, sore throats, rheumatism, inflammation and sunstroke.

Pliable blocks or slabs of tamarind are the best to work with. These blocks have been slightly fermented and therefore keep for a long time. Look for those that have not been salted. You can buy them in Asian supermarkets and increasingly in mainstream supermarkets, too. It's best to avoid the concentrated tamarind pastes you may see in the shops, as these have been further processed and usually contain preservatives; the flavour is also not as good.

You can also buy tamarind pods, but you need to peel them, press them together to form a big ball or block, and then leave on the counter to ferment for several days, until it becomes very sour.

TURMERIC 'BUG'

For making the Turmeric Cream Soda (see p. 106). This is fermented turmeric root – it becomes slightly acidic and probiotic.

UNREFINED SALTS

Look for sea salt, Himalayan salt, or black salt.

UNREFINED SUGARS

Rich in minerals and vitamins and extracted from plants and blossoms, such as:

Coconut Blossom Nectar - the thickened nectar of the coconut flower. This can be found in the sugar and sweeteners section of supermarkets and health food stores.

Honey - made by bees from blossom nectar.

Jaggery - the molasses created from the sap of sugar cane.

Maple Syrup - the sweet, thickened juice of the maple tree.

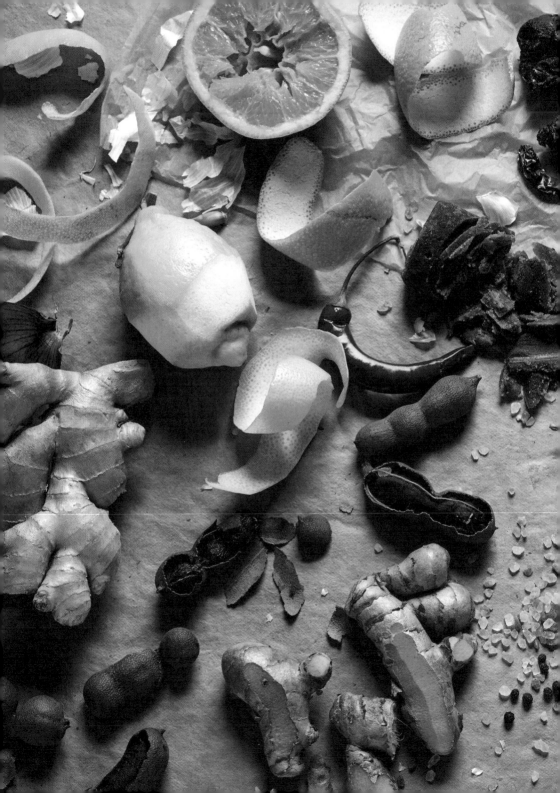

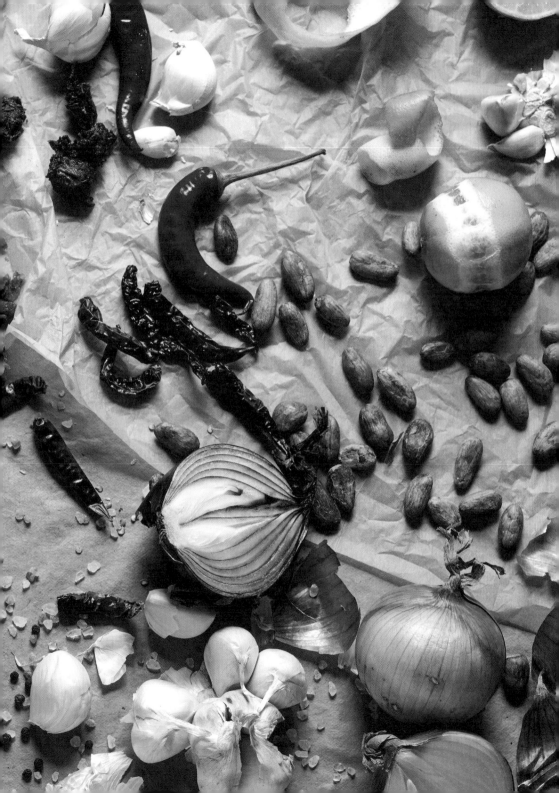

TURMERIC TAMARIND TONIC

JAMU KUNYIT ASAM

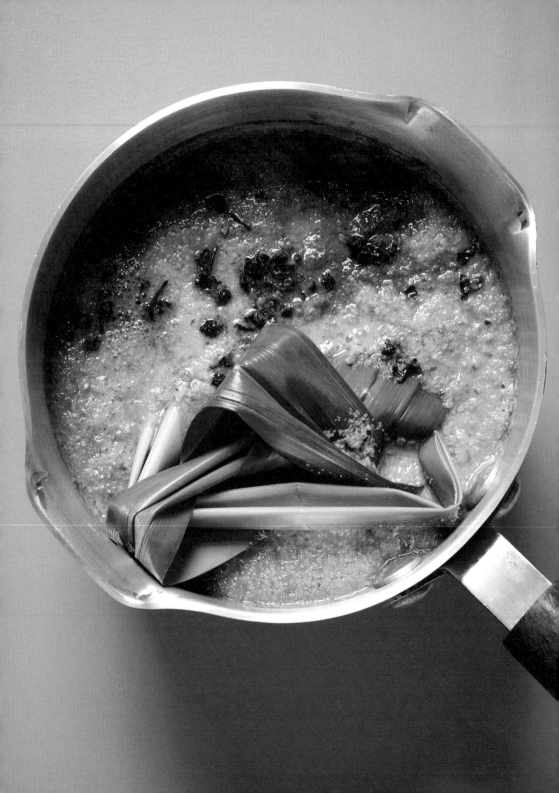

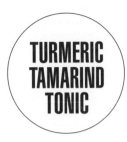

TURMERIC TAMARIND TONIC

The most popular remedy prescribed by the traditional healing system of Indonesia, known as *Jamu*, this tonic is consumed by Indonesians of all ages for its purifying, healing and beautifying powers. It is made at home according to closely-guarded family recipes, passed down from generation to generation, and humbly sold, hawker-style, to nearby neighbours and friends throughout the islands of Bali and Java. This is the very recipe I learned to make in Ubud, from the Jamu Gendong (which translates as 'Jamu carrier') herself, and inspired my journey into tonic-making. Hopefully, it will do the same for you.

Turmeric supports the liver with detoxification, purifying the blood, reducing inflammation and preventing blood clotting. Tamarind is cooling, rich in antioxidants, boosts the metabolism, suppresses the appetite and lowers blood sugar levels. As a member of the ginger family, galangal warms the body and aids in digestion.

(Recipe overleaf.)

Jamu is a 5,000-year-old system of natural healing from Indonesia, similar to Ayurveda, the traditional healing system of India. It relies solely on the power of local roots, herbs, spices and barks to cure whatever ails you.

(Continued from previous page.)

INGREDIENTS

Makes 2 litres
(70 fl oz)
Ready in 2 hours

160 g (5½ oz) fresh turmeric
root, unpeeled

40 g (1½ oz) fresh ginger
root, unpeeled

80 g (2¾ oz) seedless
tamarind block

80 g (2¾ oz/scant ½ cup)
coconut blossom nectar

a good crack of freshly
ground black pepper

pinch of sea salt

2 litres (70 fl oz)
filtered water

EQUIPMENT

large, heavy-based,
stainless-steel saucepan,
that will hold at least
2 litres (70 fl oz)

blender

plastic gloves (highly
recommended!)

fine mesh sieve (strainer)

glass measuring jug

sterilised glass bottles
(see p. 19)

glass or stainless-steel
utensils for this recipe.
Plastic will stain!

METHOD

Start by cleaning your turmeric, ginger and galangal roots (if using) roots, as we leave the skins on for this recipe. Leave them to soak in water for about 2 minutes – this helps to remove the dust that gets caught in the crevices. Then give them a good scrub and final rinse. Set aside.

Next, make the tamarind concentrate. Break up the tamarind block into very small pieces, then put them into a large, heavy-based, stainless steel saucepan, along with the coconut blossom nectar, pepper, salt and about 500 ml (17 fl oz) of the water. Place over a high heat, bring to a gentle simmer, then reduce the heat to low-medium and cook for about 20 minutes, until the tamarind has broken down to a pulp and the sugar has dissolved. Don't let it boil.

Meanwhile, it's time to blend your turmeric, ginger and galangal roots. Cut them into manageable chunks that will make them easier to blend. Add to a blender, with about 500 ml (17 fl oz) of the water, and blend to a smooth paste. You may need to add a little more water to get it as smooth as possible.

Once the tamarind pulp is ready, turn the heat under the saucepan down to low. Add the spice paste and the remaining 1 litre (35 fl oz) water. If using, tie the pandan leaf in a knot and add this to the brew. Brew for about 30 minutes, stirring every now and again.

Once ready, strain through a fine mesh sieve (strainer) into a measuring jug. You can now serve straight away or pour into sterilised glass bottles. Tightly sealed, it will keep in the fridge for up to 20 days.

You can drink the jamu hot or cold, preferably first thing in the morning on an empty stomach.

OPTIONAL EXTRAS *20g (¾ oz) fresh galangal;*
1 fresh pandan leaf (both can be found at most Asian
supermarkets)

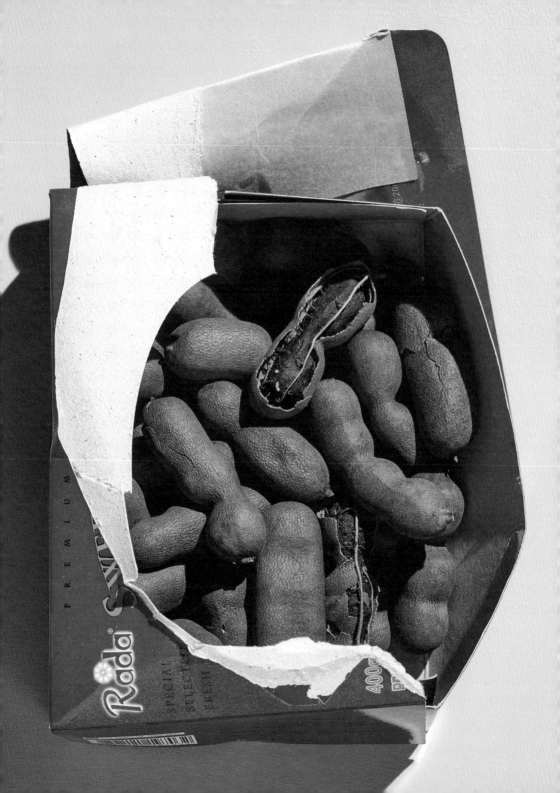

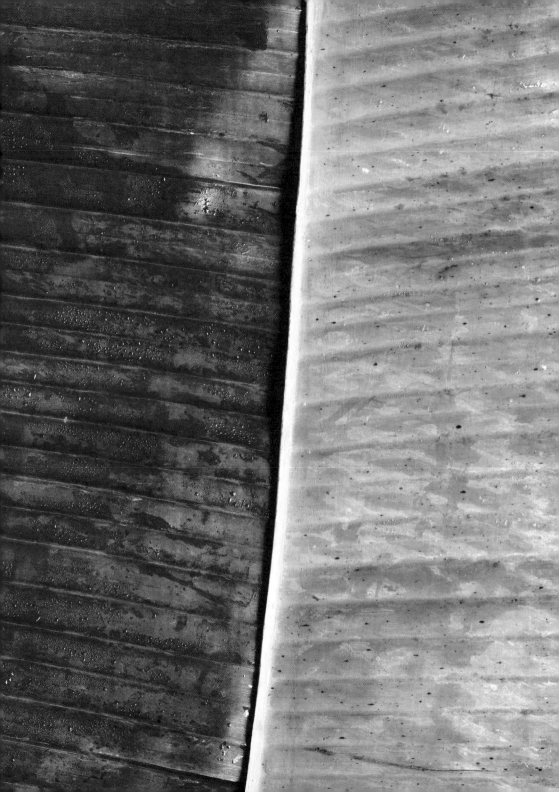

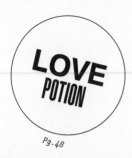

Pg.48

Chapter 1

STRESSED?

SLOW DOWN. CHILL OUT. MAKE A TONIC.

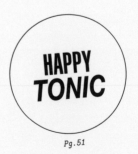

Pg.51

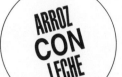

Pg. 52

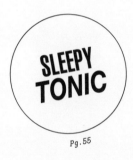

Pg. 55

Spending time in the kitchen can be therapeutic. It quiets the mind.

Mental stress has physical consequences. It builds up slowly inside, and it can take years before it becomes visible as a physical illness on the outside. Stress affects every system in the body, including our adrenal and thyroid glands, and hormones. It also ages skin, depletes energy and immunity, and compromises digestion.

Stress has the ability to reduce the diversity of your gut bacteria. The less diverse they become, the more susceptible you become to illness, food allergies and sensitivities.

No matter how hard you work on your health, until you manage your stress levels, you will never be fully well. Adopting stress-free habits will create a rock-solid foundation that will not only improve your mood, skin, hair, weight and energy levels, but can also help to slow down the ageing process. Tonic making is a form of meditation and creative expression that is rewarded with a quality drink afterwards.

This chapter is all about feeling good, from the inside out. Beauty is a state of grace, achieved when you reach your true potential for happiness, health and creativity. Balancing stress hormones is the key to truly sustainable radiance.

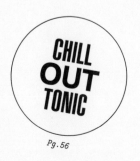

Pg. 56

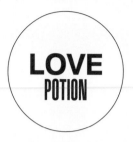

LOVE POTION

Chocolate makes you happy. Naturally occurring chemicals in this forbidden fruit can affect the human brain – consuming chocolate releases several neurotransmitters that positively affect your emotions. One of these is phenylethylamine, also known as 'the love drug', which triggers a degree of excitement, quickens the heart rate, and arouses feelings similar to those of being in love. Another neurotransmitter, serotonin, lifts your mood.

This spicy hot chocolate recipe takes things to another level, with a few warming, metabolism- and immunity-boosting spices. Cayenne pepper and cinnamon help boost the healing and 'happiness' properties of the cacao and balance out blood sugar levels.

INGREDIENTS

Makes 2 servings
Ready in 10 minutes

230 ml (7¾ fl oz) coconut milk

230 ml (7¾ fl oz) just-boiled water

4 tbsp raw cacao powder

4 squares of your favourite dark chocolate

1 tsp ground cinnamon

¼ tsp cayenne pepper

¼ tsp chilli powder

¼ tsp pink Himalayan salt

¼ tsp ground turmeric

coconut sugar or honey, to taste

METHOD

Add all the ingredients (except your sweetener) to a large saucepan and bring to a simmer over a low heat. Simmer for 2–3 minutes, whisking, until thoroughly melted and mixed together, then remove from the heat. Add your chosen sweetener, to taste, then pour into 2 mugs to serve.

A drink for two.

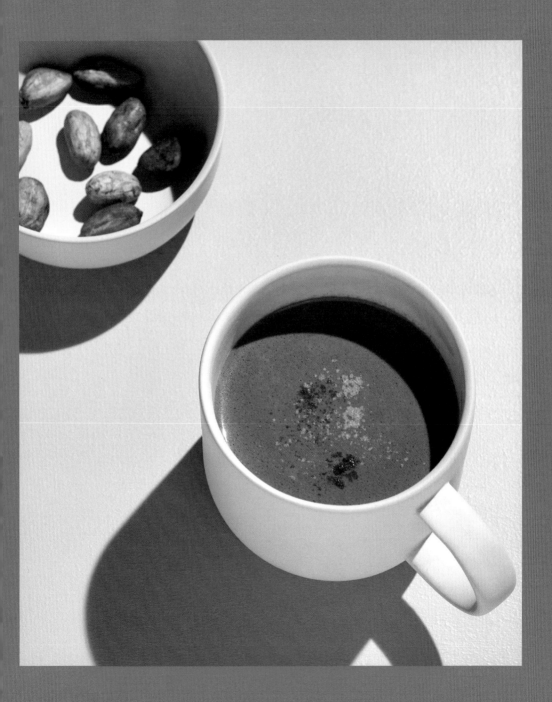

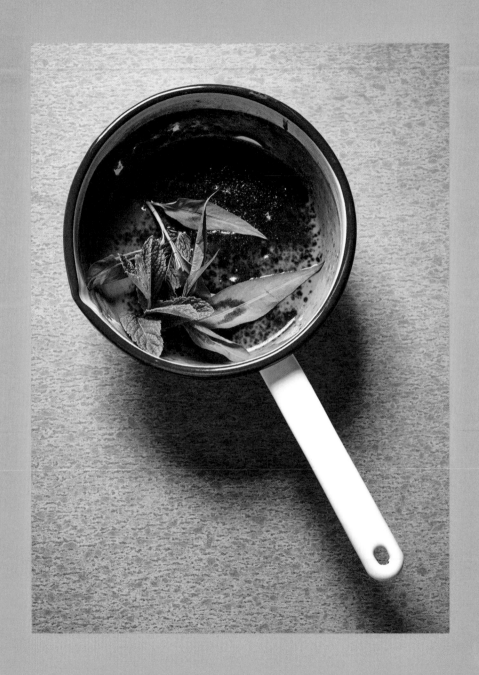

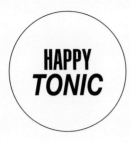

HAPPY TONIC

If chocolate makes you happy, imagine what a mint and chocolate combo can do. This tonic is well suited for after eight, or any time of day for that matter.

Mint has been used as a medicinal herb for hundreds of years. Its benefits include aiding digestion, promoting weight loss, and relieving headaches and nausea. Mint is also a natural stimulant – the smell alone can be enough to recharge your batteries. If you are feeling sluggish, anxious, depressed, or simply exhausted, mint will help to invigorate and relax you.

Fresh mint-infused hot chocolate.

INGREDIENTS

Makes 2 servings
Ready in 30 minutes

230 ml (7¾ fl oz) coconut milk

2–3 sprigs of fresh mint

230 ml (7¾ fl oz) just-boiled water

4 tbsp raw cacao powder, or 4 squares of your favourite dark chocolate

2 tbsp raw cacao nibs

1 tsp ground cinnamon

¼ tsp cayenne pepper

¼ tsp chilli powder

¼ tsp pink Himalayan salt

¼ tsp ground turmeric

Coconut sugar or honey, to taste

METHOD

In a small saucepan, bring the coconut milk to a simmer over a medium heat. Add your freshly spanked mint leaves, then turn the heat to low. Leave to gently infuse for 15 minutes, then remove from the heat and leave to cool.

Once cooled, add all the remaining ingredients (except your chosen sweetener) to the saucepan, and bring back to a simmer over a low heat, whisking thoroughly. Simmer for 2–3 minutes, then remove from the heat, add your chosen sweetener, to taste, and pour into 2 mugs to serve.

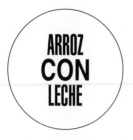

ARROZ CON LECHE

This traditional drink from Mexico, called a horchata, has the comforting starchiness and taste of the rice pudding or the Spanish 'arroz con leche' I had growing up. It is surprisingly brilliant in the summer, served cold over ice.

It's the ultimate comfort drink – made from rice, almonds and coconut, spiced with cinnamon and cloves – it also happens to be a perfect dairy-free alternative to milk.

Starchy rice water is an ancient Indonesian healing tonic that provides instant energy, improves digestion, stabilises blood sugar levels, and slows down ageing, while also providing the body with essential vitamins. Javanese housewives even save rice water to use as a face toner after cooking the family meal.

Spiced rice milk horchata.

INGREDIENTS

Makes 4 large servings
Ready in 14 hours

200 g (7 oz/1 cup plus 2 tbsp) long-grain rice

100 g (3½ oz/generous ½ cup) raw almonds

4 cinnamon sticks or 2 tsp ground cinnamon

4 whole cloves or a pinch of ground cloves

850 ml (30 fl oz) water

½ x 330 ml (11 fl oz) tin coconut milk, to taste

coconut blossom nectar, to taste

METHOD

Start the night before. In a large frying pan (skillet), toast the rice over a medium heat, stirring, until fragrant and golden – about 25 minutes. Remove from the heat and let the rice cool completely before moving on to the next stage – you don't want it to cook.

Rinse the cooled rice under cold water. Transfer it to a large bowl and add the almonds, cinnamon, cloves and water. Cover and leave it to soak overnight in 850 ml (30 fl oz) water.

The next day, transfer the mixture to a blender and pulse 2–3 times, just enough to break up the rice a little – you don't want to completely pulverise it.

Strain through a fine mesh sieve or muslin (cheesecloth) – you may need to do this a few times. At this point, you should have a very basic rice milk.

Add coconut milk and coconut blossom nectar, to taste. Whisk thoroughly until the texture is smooth. Refrigerate until cold, before serving.

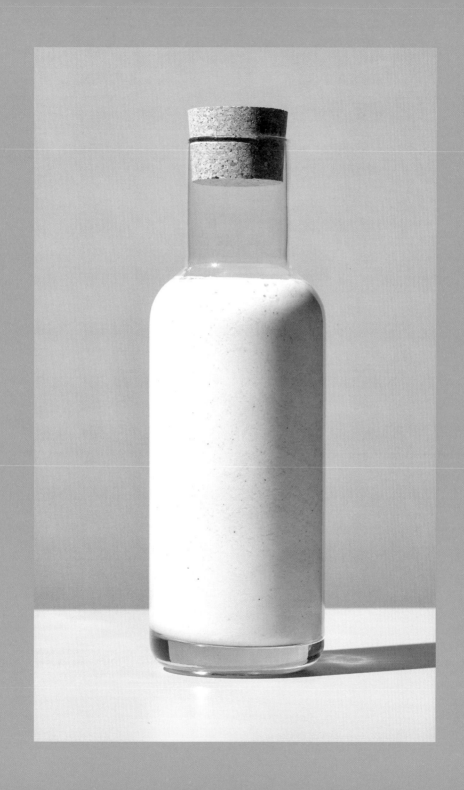

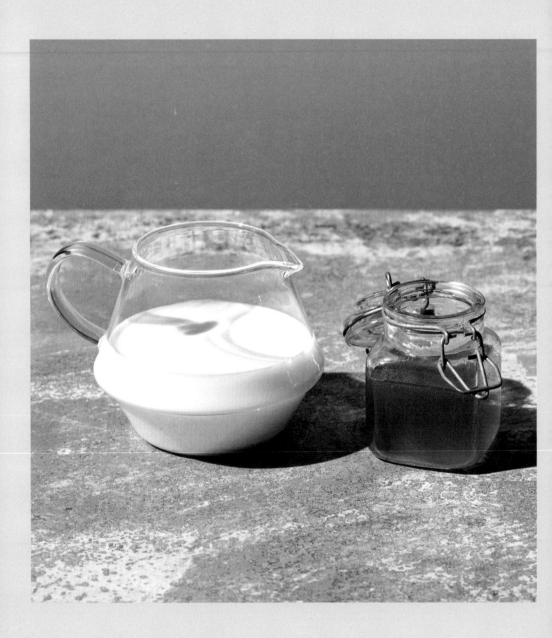

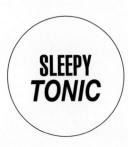

SLEEPY TONIC

A recipe inspired by my childhood. *Anijsmelk* (aniseed milk) is an old-fashioned Dutch nightcap. The warmth of the milk, and the soothing flavours and benefits of aniseed, honey and sesame, work wonders for the stomach and the mind.

Drinking hot milk before bed has been used a sleep remedy for thousands of years across Europe and in Ayurvedic medicine. The bioactive peptides in milk, when taken before bed, have been scientifically proven to improve sleep, which means that your mother was right about it being a powerful sleep medicine after all. If you're dairy intolerant, feel free to use any other 'milk' that suits you best (although I can't guarantee its effectiveness).

Milk and honey.

INGREDIENTS

Makes 1 serving
Ready in 10 minutes

1 tbsp of aniseed (anise) (optional)

1 tbsp of black sesame seeds (optional)

250 ml (9 fl oz) non-homogenised organic milk

honey or Fermented Honey (see p. 144), to taste

METHOD

To prepare your sleep aid, blend the aniseed and black sesame seeds (if using) with a dash of milk in a blender, to create a paste. You can also use a pestle and mortar.

Place all of the ingredients (including the paste, if making) in a saucepan and warm through over a gentle heat until hot. Add honey of choice, to taste, and strain before serving.

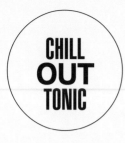

CHILL OUT TONIC

This tasty homemade peanut milk is an option for those seeking to chill their beans. It's an alternative nut milk, like no other.

Peanuts, despite what anybody's told you, aren't actually nuts, they're legumes – a class of vegetables that includes beans. (So glad we cleared that up.) Peanuts are also a comfort food. They contain substances that activate neurotransmitters, or brain chemicals, that stabilise your mood. Which means that the emotional and physical responses you get from drinking peanut milk could actually help you deal with anxiety.

Roasted peanut milk.

INGREDIENTS

Makes 4 large servings
Ready in 14 hours

135 g (4¾ oz/1 cup) raw peanuts, skins on

pinch of sea salt

1 tbsp coconut blossom nectar, to taste

350 ml (12 fl oz) filtered water

METHOD

Start the night before. Spread the peanuts out on a baking tray (shallow baking pan) and roast in the oven at 180°C (350° F/Gas 4), for about 20–25 minutes, until they are light golden brown (keep your eye on them and take them out of the oven as soon as they turn golden as they will keep cooking as they cool). Then, leave them to soak in water overnight.

The next day, drain and rinse the peanuts thoroughly. Place the soaked peanuts into a high-powered blender, with the salt and coconut blossom nectar, and add the filtered water. Blend until smooth.

Pour the mixture into a nut milk bag set over a bowl. Squeeze, to get out as much liquid as you can. Transfer your peanut milk to a storage container and keep in the fridge for up to 3 days.

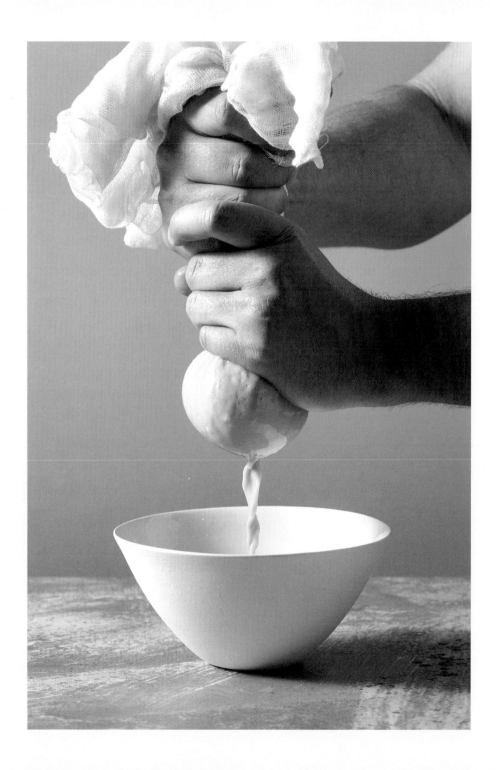

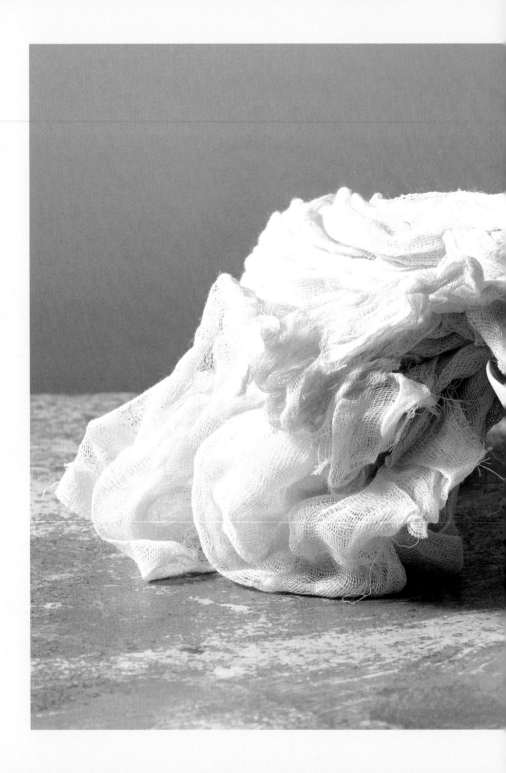

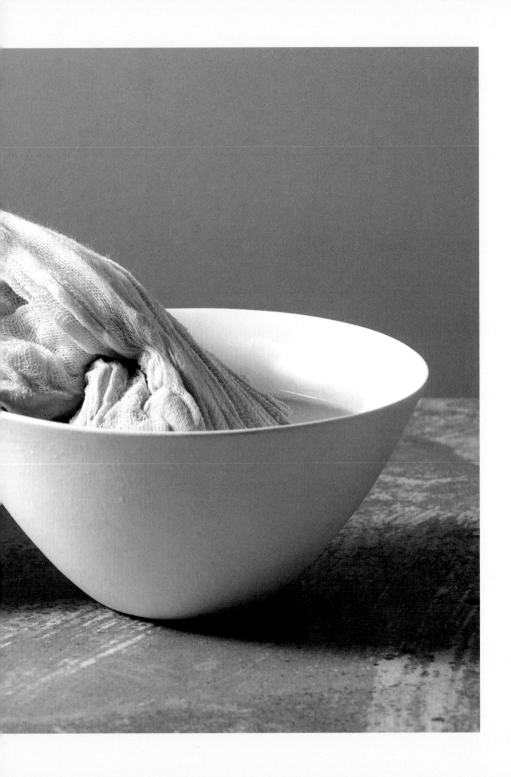

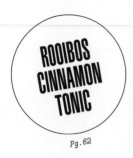

Pg. 62

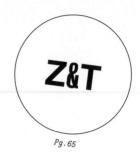

Pg. 65

Chapter 2

TIRED?

SHAKE UP YOUR WAKE UP.
GET ENERGISED.
WITH AN ENERGY TONIC.

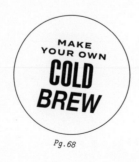

Pg. 68

There's absolutely nothing wrong with tea or coffee. In fact, there's a lot to love about a magical leaf or bean that gives you energy, among other very legit health benefits.

Having said that, there are times when your regular flat white or afternoon cup of builder's brew just isn't on the cards, because it's making you crash, anxious or keeping you up at night. Caffeine is, after all, a stimulant. Although drinking it drowns out our symptoms of tiredness, it's merely a quick fix. It puts our energy levels on a constant rollercoaster of highs and lows. This will only make you more tired in the long run. It drains you, and then you get ill.

Cutting down on caffeine, or finding new varieties and ways of preparing your morning brew that have less imposing effects on the balance of your system, will ultimately help to increase energy levels.

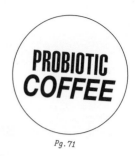

PROBIOTIC COFFEE

Pg. 71

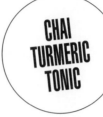

CHAI TURMERIC TONIC

Pg. 72

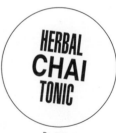

HERBAL CHAI TONIC

Pg. 73

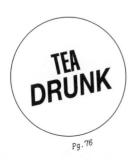

TEA DRUNK

Pg. 76

This chapter is about discovering new, sustainable ways to wake you up without cracking you out. Breaking habits is very hard to do, so in times like these, it's nice to have a few options that are equally hot (some cold), steamy (or refreshing) and, of course, energising.

Here are my favourites, some non-caffeinated and some subtly so.

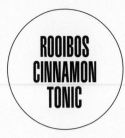

ROOIBOS CINNAMON TONIC

A rooibos (pronounced roy-boss) latte is deliciously nutty and satisfying – perfect for those seeking a caffeine-free alternative to coffee.

This red tea is loaded with antioxidants. It has anti-inflammatory and antifungal properties; helps with nervous tension and headaches, skin problems and digestive complaints; and it also boosts the immune system.

Rooibos is a medicinal herb that is acquired from an indigenous red bush plant, which grows only in the mountainous region of Cape Town. It's been a favourite among South Africans for hundreds of years.

Naturally caffeine-free.

INGREDIENTS

Makes 4 servings
Ready in 15 minutes

5 tsp rooibos (red bush) tea leaves

½ a cinnamon stick

200 ml (7 fl oz) just-boiled water

800 ml (28 fl oz) milk of choice

1 tsp of honey or coconut sugar

METHOD

Make a rooibos concentrate by brewing the tea and cinnamon in just-boiled water for 10 minutes. It needs to be nice and strong.

Meanwhile, heat the milk in a saucepan over a gentle heat.

When ready, strain the rooibos tea and stir in a teaspoon of sweetener. Divide between 4 glasses or mugs and pour the hot milk over each. Serve immediately.

Keep any leftover concentrate in the fridge for up to 3 days.

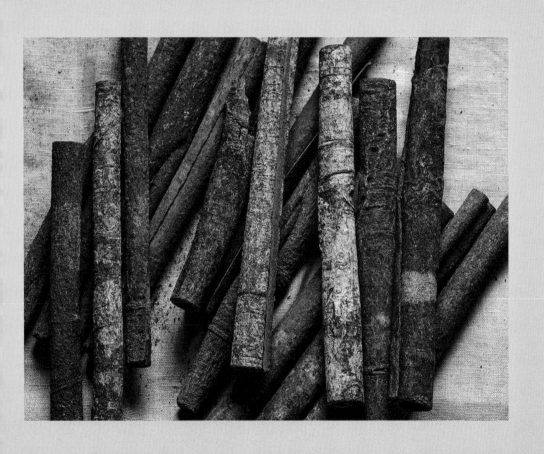

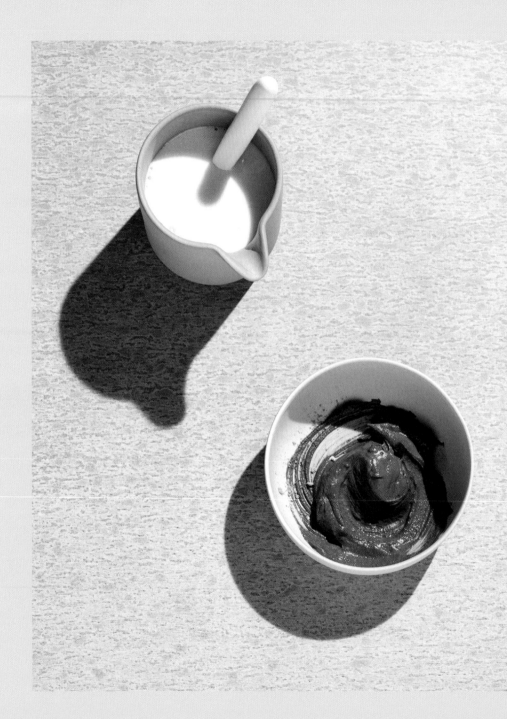

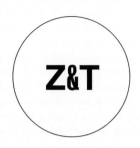

Z&T

A cup of matcha (ground green tea) stimulates both mental alertness, and a calm, meditative state of mind, without any of the nervous energy some get from regular coffee. Combined with soy milk – a traditional Chinese staple – this is the perfect energy tonic.

Matcha originated in China during the Tang dynasty (618–907 AD). A monk named Eisai introduced both the Zen philosophy and matcha tea to Japan in 1191 – he was the first person to grind and consume the entire tea-leaf in powdered form. Eisai would drink matcha during long hours of meditating, to remain alert yet calm. As a result, Zen and matcha became inextricably linked in the form of a sacred tea ceremony. This ceremony celebrates the profound beauty of simple things, the extraordinary in the ordinary, and aims to bring participants into the here and now.

Matcha with homemade almond soy milk.

INGREDIENTS

*Makes about 750 ml
(26 fl oz)
Ready in 11 hours*

For the 'milk'

170 g (6 oz/1 generous cup)
dried soya beans (soybeans)

6 raw almonds

1 litre (35 fl oz)
filtered water

For the tea

matcha tea powder
(1 heaped tsp per cup)

Honey or sweetener of
choice (optional)

METHOD

Start the night before, Soak the soybeans and almonds overnight, or for at least 10 hours, at room temperature.

Drain, then transfer the soaked beans and nuts to a blender, add the filtered water, and blend until smooth.

Strain the mixture through a muslin (cheesecloth) twice, to filter out all the fibre and create a smooth 'milk'. This will last in the fridge for several days, and can also be frozen.

Once ready to drink, transfer the 'milk', as needed, to a heavy-based saucepan and simmer on a low heat for 10 minutes. You'll need about 250 ml (9 fl oz) per cup.

Once hot, whisk the matcha into the 'milk', until smooth and clump-free. Sweeten, if desired, and serve.

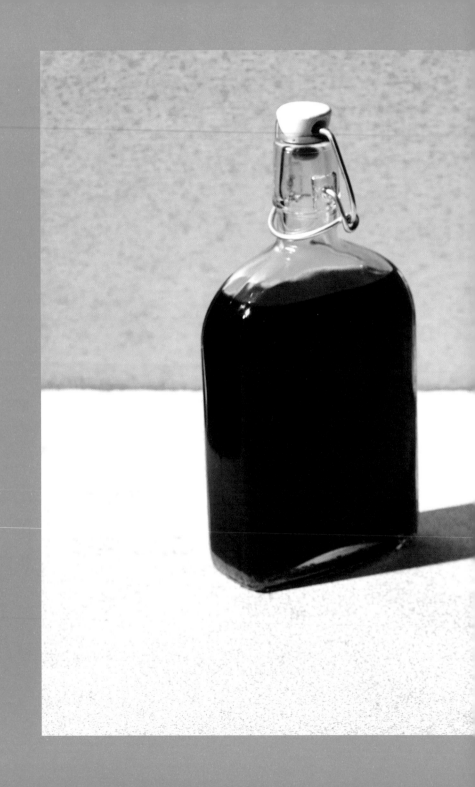

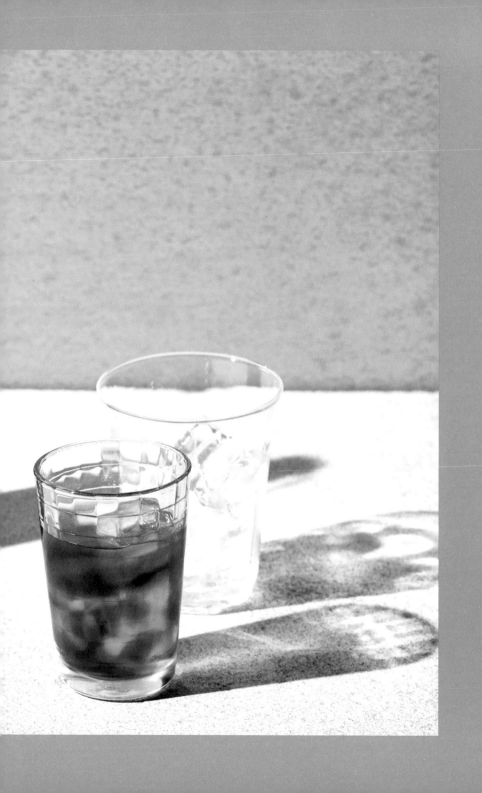

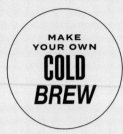

MAKE YOUR OWN COLD BREW

Coffee extracted in cold water is the most refreshing coffee drink on earth. It goes down easy, but be warned: it is highly caffeinated. The benefit of cold brew is that it is much less acidic than typical hot-brewed coffee. It's also smoother and less bitter in flavour, giving it a tonic-like quality.

The first evidence of true cold-brewed coffee (or Kyoto-style coffee), made with cold water, comes from Japan. Records show that the Japanese have been brewing coffee this way for at least four centuries.

Even the traditional system of Jamu recommends steeping coffee cold overnight, to avoid disturbing sensitive stomachs.

A guide by Luke Suddards, co-founder of Sandows in London.

INGREDIENTS

*Makes 1 litre
(35 fl oz)
Ready in 12-24 houra*

70 g (2½ oz/1 scant cup) fresh coarsely ground coffee

1 litre (35 fl oz) cold water

METHOD

Start the day before. Place the freshly ground coffee and the water into the container and stir until the coffee is well soaked. Cover and place in the fridge for 12–24 hours. I usually steep mine for around 16 hours, but it's worth playing around to see if you like it stronger or weaker.

Once steeped, and trying not to disturb the ground coffee at the bottom, either decant your cold brew into a French press and plunge, or pour it through a filter paper, before serving over ice.

It will keep in the fridge for up to 4 weeks.

For the tastiest brew, grind the coffee just before you steep it and use spring water if you're in a hard water area. I like to use a medium to light roast to let more of the delicate flavours shine. I always recommend to use filter papers if possible, for a cleaner, clearer brew, but a cafetiere (French Press) will also give great results and is much more likely to be in the cupboard.

EQUIPMENT

Coffee grinder

Large container

Filter papers or a French press (cafetiere)

COMBINATIONS

Cardamom and Vanilla Cold Brew
Infuse your brew with a little spice. Once you've placed your coffee into your container, add the 3 cardamom pods and ½ a vanilla pod. Steep for 16 hours in the fridge, as before.

Cold Brew and Tonic
An oddball combination – but that's ok. Drop a splash of your cold brew into a glass of tonic water over ice and twist some orange peel into it for a zesty touch. Add gin too if it's Friday!

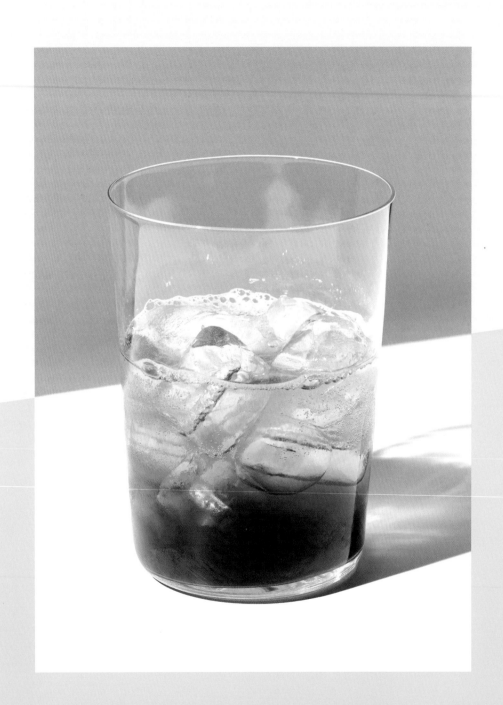

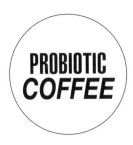

PROBIOTIC COFFEE

This is a take on the unbeatable combination of iced tea and lemonade. Made with cold-brewed coffee and kombucha – it's a coffee on tea paradox.

Coffee combined with a healthy dose of kombucha's probiotics creates a surprisingly flavoursome and thirst quenching energy tonic that is refreshing and invigorating at the same time.

Iced coffee with a fermented twist.

INGREDIENTS

Makes 4 servings
Ready in 5 minutes

1 litres (35 fl oz) of Cold Brew coffee (see p. 68)

1 lemon, sliced

ice, to serve

1 litre (35 fl oz) shop-bought kombucha (or see p. 118 to make your own lemon-flavoured booch)

METHOD

Slice the lemon, add to a glass and fill it to the top with ice. Fill the glass half way with the kombucha, then top up with the cold brewed coffee. Mix and enjoy.

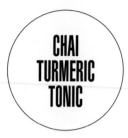

CHAI TURMERIC TONIC

This Chai is a spicy and invigorating blend of medicinally active spices such as turmeric, ginger, cloves, cinnamon, cardamom, nutmeg and black pepper. Chai can be a personal thing, so feel free to use this recipe as a guideline to find your perfect brew – adjust it to suit your sassiness.

This complex concoction not only wakes you up, it calms the mind, improves digestion, enhances the immune system, fights inflammation and is loaded with antioxidants.

Chai has been cherished in Indian households for centuries. Grandma – the household caretaker – would brew a blend of plant roots, bark and seeds if a family member became ill or as a tonic to stay healthy through the changing seasons. Eventually, tea, with its energy-giving medicinal properties, made its way into Grandma's spice tonic, and made chai what it is today.

INGREDIENTS

Makes 1 serving
Ready in 10 minutes

2 black peppercorns

2 green cardamom pods

1 clove

½ a cinnamon stick

1 black tea bag or 1 tbsp black loose leaf tea

a few slices of fresh ginger root

a few slices of fresh turmeric root

120 ml (4 fl oz) water

120 ml (4 fl oz) milk of choice

sweetener of choice

METHOD

In a frying pan (skillet) set over a medium heat, dry roast your peppercorns, cardamom pods, clove, and cinnamon stick until they become aromatic, then lightly crush them with a pestle and mortar.

Blend your slices of ginger and turmeric with a little bit of water in a blender to make a paste. You could also grate them. Or mash them in a pestle and mortar.

In a saucepan set over a medium heat, add the water, ginger and turmeric paste, tea and crushed spices. Bring to a boil, then reduce the heat to low and simmer for 5 minutes.

Add the milk and sweetener to taste. Turn the heat up to medium, and bring the mixture back to a boil. Remove from the heat and strain into a mug, to serve.

The sassiest cup of builder's brew.

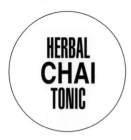

HERBAL CHAI TONIC

Chai infused with perky lemongrass and mint.

This recipe is designed for that transitional time of year when the lingering summer warmth starts to fade and the need for a warming yet reviving beverage starts to resurface.

The scent of herbs alone can be incredibly energising. Lemongrass paired with mint creates a clean and crisp aroma that has a powerful purifying, refreshing and energising effect on the body.

Chai infused with perky lemongrass and mint.

INGREDIENTS

Makes 1 serving
Ready in 10 minutes

2 black peppercorns

2 green cardamom pods

1 clove

½ a cinnamon stick

1 black tea bag or 1 tbsp black loose leaf tea

a few slices of fresh ginger root

5 fresh mint leaves

1 lemongrass

120 ml (4 fl oz) water

120 ml (4 fl oz) milk of choice

sweetener of choice

METHOD

Follow the Chai Turmeric Tonic recipe (see opposite), but leave out the turmeric. There's no need to make a ginger paste either, just slice it finely. Instead of turmeric, we're going to add fresh mint and lemongrass.

Spank the mint leaves, and bruise the white end of the lemongrass, with the flat side of a cleaver or pestle, and cut into thin slices.

Add them to your saucepan, along with all your chai spices and tea and brew on a low heat as usual. Remove from the heat and strain into a mug, to serve.

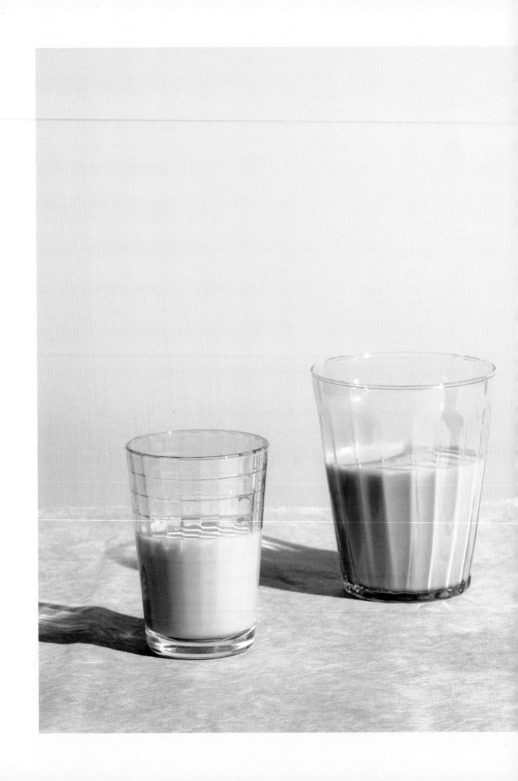

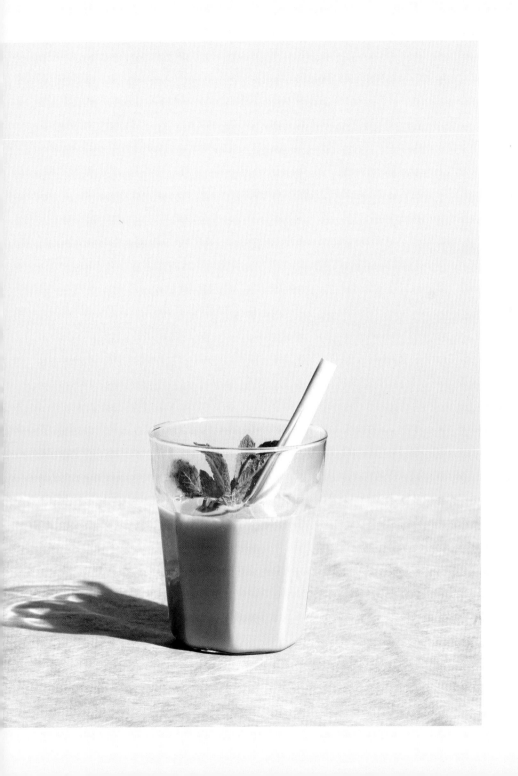

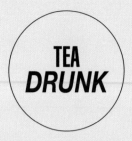

TEA DRUNK

Being 'tea drunk' is a legitimate thing in China. It's known as "cha zui". When done right, it can feel euphoric. I feel focused, calm, content, and perhaps even a little giggly. I also feel contemplative, introspective and philosophical. All in all, the effect is very 'zen'.

The physical, mental and emotional effects of tea give me more reasons to love it. Being drunk on tea is the result of the combination of caffeine and other molecules in tea, particularly L-theanine. L-theanine induces a very calm, yet sleepy, state, which can ease anxiety. However, when you combine it with caffeine, L-theanine increases the production of alpha waves in the brain, inducing a meditative state without making you tired.

Lining the stomach with some food before getting 'tea drunk' is highly recommended. Otherwise side effects such as shakiness, nausea, dizziness and other unpleasant stuff associated with drinking too much caffeine could occur.

Ironically, getting drunk on tea, particularly green tea, is traditionally believed to be a good cure for a hangover by the Chinese and Japanese.

You can only get tea drunk by drinking the high-quality stuff, by the way.

TEA

All teas, apart from herbal teas, are produced from the same plant, known as *Camellia sinensis*. Each type has different processing methods, aromas, flavours and benefits that set it apart from the rest. Drinking this tea leaf improves hydration, focus and concentration, and helps maintain a positive mood throughout the day. Look for loose-leaf, premium-grade teas.

Black (fermented) This tea is made from leaves that have been fully fermented. The leaf is spread out and left to wilt naturally, before being roasted, producing a deep, rich flavour and an amber brew.

Blue-green (semi-fermented)
Oolong (pronounced 'wu long') falls right in-between green and black tea. It's gently rolled after picking and allowed to partially ferment, until the edges of the leaves start to turn brown. It has a natural ability to aid weight loss. Foodies, wine fanatics and serious tea drinkers boast about its incredible depth and complexity – making it the connoisseur's tea of choice.

Green (roasted/steamed) Packed with high levels of antioxidants, green tea is withered, then steamed or heated to prevent oxidation, then rolled and dried. It is characterized by a delicate taste and light green colour.

While green teas are available almost everywhere, these tend to be low quality. If your current brand of green tea is simply called 'green tea', it probably isn't of a very good quality. Look for 'types' of green tea, such as:

Japanese Sencha – this makes an especially good kombucha.

Genmaicha – Sencha mixed with toasted rice.

Hojicha – roasted Sencha.

Shincha – made from 'new' green tea leaves, usually the first picking of the season. These new leaves have a distinctly refreshing and invigorating scent, and contain a lot less caffeine too.

Matcha (ground green tea) Matcha is the entire leaf in powdered form, made from stoneground Tencha tea, which makes it the most potent way to ingest green tea. Matcha is rich in antioxidants and L-Theanine, a rare amino acid that actually promotes a state of relaxation and wellbeing by influencing brain function.

White (sun-dried) The rarest and most delicate of teas. White tea is plucked and simply air-dried in the sun, which preserves even more of its antioxidant properties.

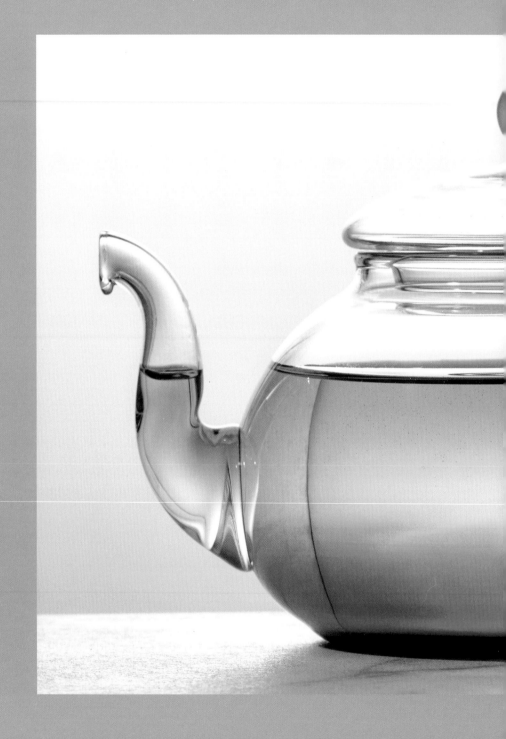

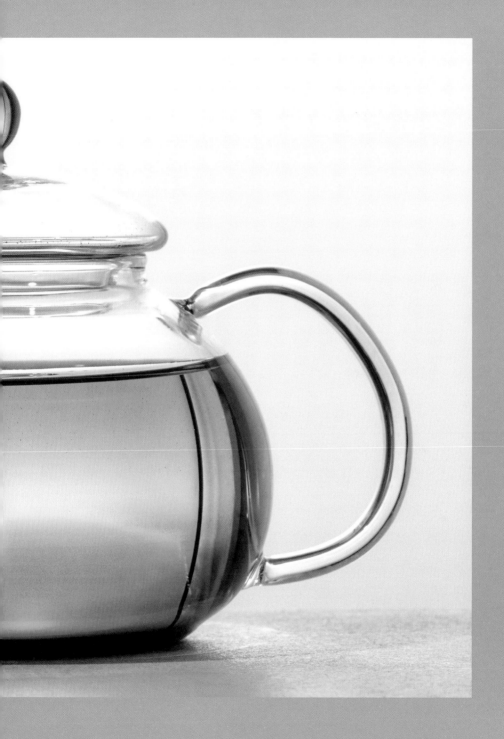

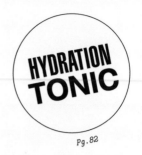

HYDRATION TONIC

Pg.82

Chapter 3

HUNGOVER?

THIS CHAPTER IS ABOUT FEELING ABSOLUTELY TERRIBLE. SURVIVING. SURVIVAL TONICS.

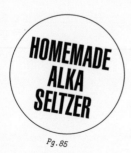

HOMEMADE ALKA SELTZER

Pg.85

Unfortunately there are no shortcuts, or miracle cures here – only time can reduce the level of alcohol in your body. The way you spend this time, though, can certainly help the process. Spend a good part of the day on yourself and your 'condition'. Make a tonic.

This chapter offers a few dead simple remedies to help get you through, as well as a few elaborate recipes to help distract the mind from the guilt, and shame – hangovers truly are a mind and body experience like no other.

These survival or hangover tonics incorporate the liver-supportive herbs and spices you need to lower your toxic load, but are also down-to-earth (and tasty) enough to enjoy when you're back to 'normal'. There's no need to endure any more suffering.

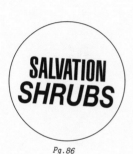

Pg.86

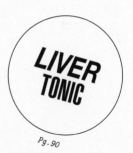

Pg.90

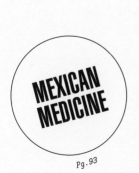

Pg.93

Start with hydration. Go beyond water. Replenish and rehydrate to kick-start the recovery process and eliminate any excess toxins. Lose the meds – they irritate the stomach and can cause liver damage when taken in excess.

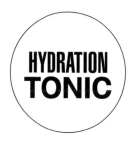

HYDRATION TONIC

Tropical relief for times of need. This tonic is thirst quenching, revitalising, nourishing, and helps sweat out nasty toxins.

Many Indians swear by coconut water as a hangover cure. Coconut water is rich in electrolytes, which means it helps replenish minerals such as potassium, salts, and fluids – perfect for helping out an already exhausted liver and restoring dehydrated and tired-looking skin too. Its cooling properties help to calm and ground anxious, heated thoughts, also known as 'the fear'.

Coconut water with lime, ginger and cardamom.

INGREDIENTS

Makes 1 serving
Ready in 5 minutes

2 fresh green
cardamom pods

1 cm (½ in) piece
of fresh ginger root

the water from
1 fresh young coconut

¼ of a lime, sliced

METHOD

In a frying pan (skillet) set over a medium heat, dry-toast the cardamom until it becomes fragrant.

In a pestle and mortar, grind the cardamom and ginger to a paste. Mix all the ingredients together in a glass and chill before serving.

For a highly sensible snack, spoon out the white coconut meat. It's loaded with good fats to help keep a ferocious appetite at bay. Delicious too.

OPTIONAL *a few drops of digestive bitters (see p. 110) and sunglasses*

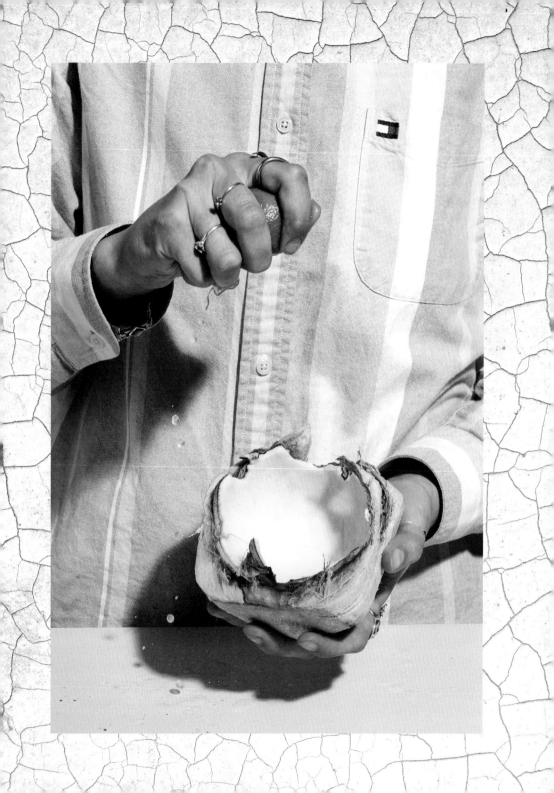

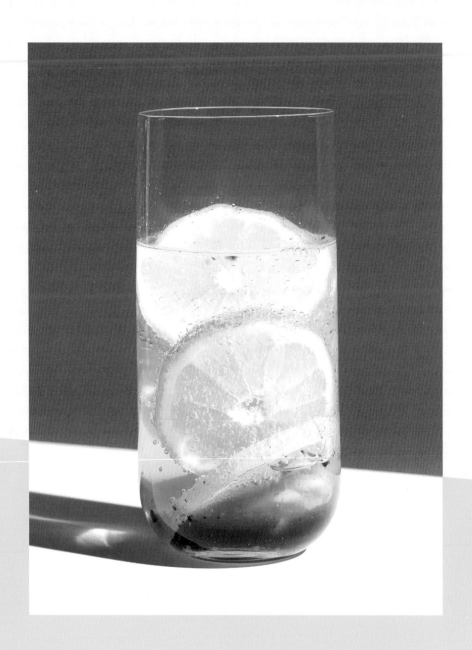

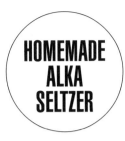

HOMEMADE ALKA SELTZER

A capable concoction, designed to come to your aid – swiftly. Do you have ginger? Do you have lemon? Great, you're almost there. All we're doing here is adding a few good sugars, salts and spices to water.

Hydrating with water alone, when your electrolytes and minerals are depleted, is simply not enough. Fresh ginger combined with the alkalinity of a lemon or lime will help settle a queasy belly by neutralising stomach acid.

'Plop-plop, fizz-fizz, oh what a relief it is.'

INGREDIENTS

Makes 1 serving
Ready in 5 minutes

300 ml (10½ fl oz) still or sparkling water

juice of 1 lemon or lime

1-cm (½-in) piece of fresh ginger root, grated

½ tsp maple syrup

pinch of sea salt

freshly ground black pepper, to taste

METHOD

Add all ingredients to a glass, then stir until the syrup and salt have dissolved.

Serve at room temperature.

OPTIONAL *a splash of digestive bitters (see p. 110)*

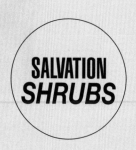

SALVATION SHRUBS

INGREDIENTS

Makes approximately
450 ml (16 fl oz)
of shrub
Ready in 2 days

450 g (1 lb) mashed fruit/
herbs/spices (75% fruit,
25% herbs and spices)

300 g (10½ oz/1½ packed
cups) unrefined sugar
(see notes below)

300 ml (10½ fl oz) vinegar
(see notes opposite)

METHOD

Start two days before. Toss your fruit, herbs, spices and peels
with sugar in a bowl or grind in a pestle and mortar. If you're using
citrus, zest the peel first and use your fingers to rub the zest
into the sugar, until it's really fragrant. Then, just chop up the
fruit, tossing it together with the zesty sugar. The same goes for
herbs – it helps to spank them first.

Let the mixture stand, covered with a tea towel (dish towel), on
your kitchen counter for approximately 2 days. Stir it once a day.

By day 2, it should look very juicy. Strain the mixture into a
measuring cup, and discard the pulp.

Then, combine your syrup with approximately an equal amount
of vinegar. Do this part slowly, tasting as you go, so that you get
a shrub that is just sharp enough, especially when using zingier
ingredients.

Pour it into a sterilised jar (see p. 19) and store it in the fridge.
It should last a few months.

Shrubs are essentially sweet and sour cordials, made by macerating whatever surplus fruit is to hand with sugar, before passing through a sieve, then adding vinegar.

Cider vinegar has a natural ability to rebalance the blood's pH level, due to its natural acidity, which helps to alkalinize the body. The reasoning behind this is that when you give your stomach more acid, it will react by needing more alkalinity, and proceed to neutralise itself. Clever stuff.

Drinking vinegars, or 'shrubs', are a tipple as old as time. Back in 17th-century England, shrubs were a way to preserve surplus fruit. The ancient Roman army added a concoction of vinegar, honey and herbs to water to make it more palatable (*posca*). Even the father of modern medicine, Hippocrates, prescribed apple cider vinegar for countless ailments.

Making the perfect shrub is all a matter of ratio. The 'sweet spot' is a 1:1:1 ratio of fruit, sugar, and vinegar.

(Recipe continued overleaf.)

NOTES ON FRUIT

I prefer my drinks a little more on the sour side, so I tend to reduce the fruit content, and replace it with more fresh roots, herbs and spices instead.

NOTES ON SUGAR

Experimenting with different kinds of good sugars, such as honey, coconut blossom nectar, jaggery, or maple syrup will add another element of flavour.

NOTES ON VINEGAR

Apple cider vinegar is a great all-rounder, but any other unpasteurised vinegar will work too.

Vinegar drinks for desperate times.

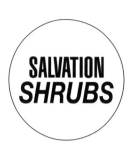

SALVATION *SHRUBS*

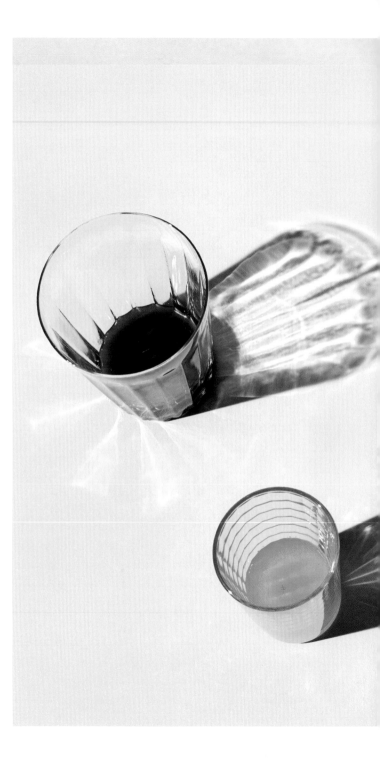

TASTY COMBINATIONS:

cucumber + dill + maple syrup + apple cider vinegar

Thai basil + lime + coconut blossom nectar + coconut vinegar

ginger + shiso leaf + honey + apple cider vinegar

turmeric + orange + black pepper + honey + apple cider vinegar

cherries + bay leaf + black pepper + maple syrup + balsamic vinegar

tomato + cardamom + lemon + lime + lemongrass + coconut blossom nectar + apple cider vinegar

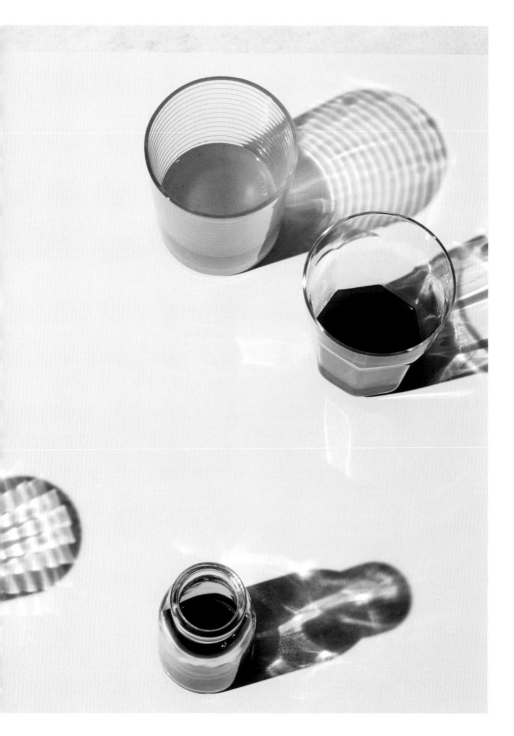

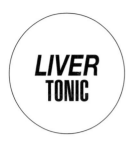

LIVER TONIC

Feeding your body with supportive herbs and spices is a brilliant way to give your liver a helping hand. Turmeric is a powerful liver-cleansing spice, with some highly potent anti-inflammatory benefits as well – incorporate it into your diet on a regular basis.

A rescue remedy: instant turmeric and ginger tonic.

INGREDIENTS

Makes 2 servings
Ready in 5 minutes

5 x 5 cm (2 in) pieces
of fresh ginger root

2 x 5 cm (2-in) pieces
of fresh turmeric root or
½ tsp ground turmeric

5 heaped tbsp honey or
Fermented Honey
(see p. 144)

juice of 1 fresh lime or lemon

2 tsp black
peppercorns

600 ml (21 fl oz) water

METHOD

Add all the ingredients to a blender and blend until smooth. Strain through a fine-mesh sieve into a large jug (pitcher) or jar.

Add a dash of bitters to serve, if desired. Garnish with mint leaves, if you're feeling fancy.

OPTIONAL *splash of homemade digestive bitters (see p. 110); fresh mint leaves, to serve*

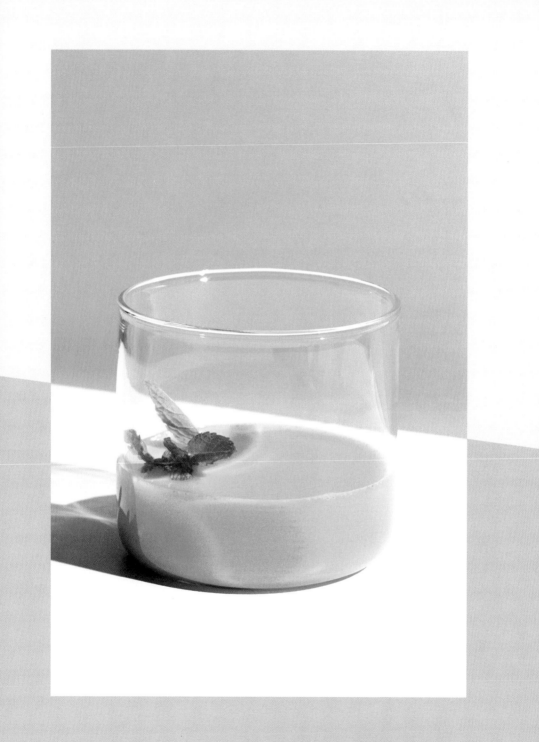

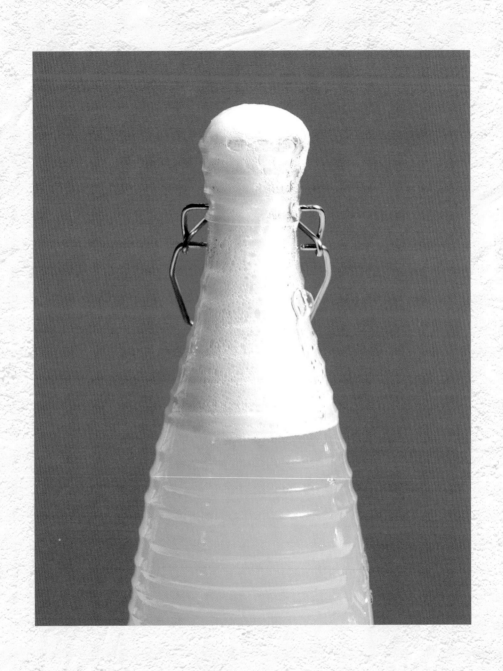

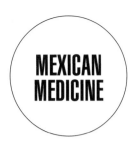

MEXICAN MEDICINE

Tepache is made using pineapple leftovers, such as the core and rinds, which are fermented with water and spices and unrefined sugar until the brew starts to fizz and develop a funky pineapple flavour. Refreshing, spicy, and a teeny touch boozy; it's perfect for soothing a hangover, and brimming with anti-inflammatory spices and natural probiotics to boost your gut health along the way. Tepache has been sold on the streets of Mexico since pre-Columbian times.

If you've decided to buy a pineapple especially for this occasion, you can use the whole fruit – just cut the skin off and eat the fruit for breakfast. The idea is that this tonic makes full use of the 'waste'.

Pineapple tepache tonic.

INGREDIENTS

Makes 2 litres (70 fl oz)
Ready in approx. 5 days

5 cloves

3-cm (1-inch) piece of fresh ginger root, bruised

5 allspice berries (optional)

2 cinnamon sticks, cracked

1 overripe pineapple, peeled and cored (save all the waste, including the leaves)

2 litres (70 fl oz) filtered water

70 g (2½ oz/⅓ cup) rapadura sugar or raw cane sugar

Lime slice, sea salt, cayenne pepper, if desired

METHOD

In a frying pan (skillet) set over a medium heat, dry-toast the spices, until they become aromatic.

Put the rinsed pineapple waste (leaves, core and rind) and spices into a large, 3-litre (105 fl oz) glass container or jug (pitcher) and add enough water to fill the remaining space.

Cover the container or jug partially – with a muslin (cheesecloth) or some loose-fitting clingfilm (plastic wrap), or simply leave the lid slightly ajar – and leave it in a warm place for 2–3 days. The rate of fermentation will depend on how warm it is. When it is near fermentation, the top of the liquid should be frothy. Scoop off the froth with a wooden spoon.

After 2–3 days, add the sugar, and loosely cover again. Feel free to reduce the sugar content a little, for a more tart flavour. Let it stand for 2 more days.

Once it's ready, strain (discard the pulp), and store in sterilised bottles (see p. 19) in the fridge. It will continue to ferment and fizz, so remember to 'burp' it (open to release the pressure) at least once a day.

Serve it ice-cold with lime, salt and a sprinkle of cayenne pepper. If you're really feeling worse for wear, do as the Mexicans do, and top it all off with a good glug of beer.

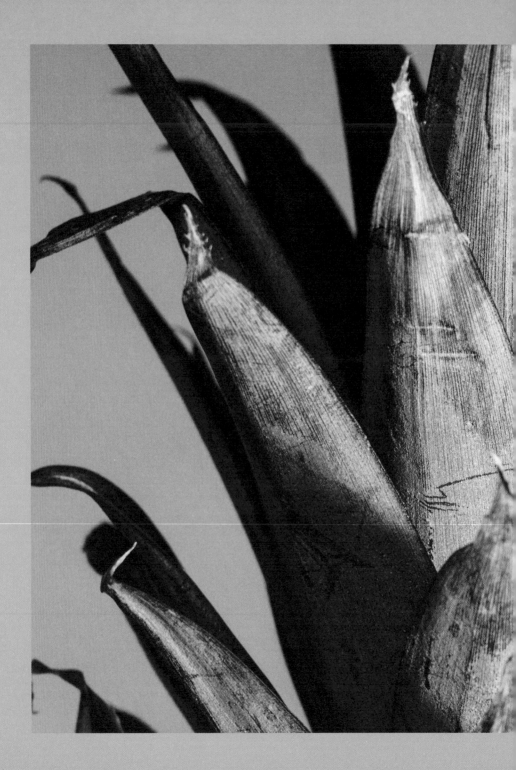

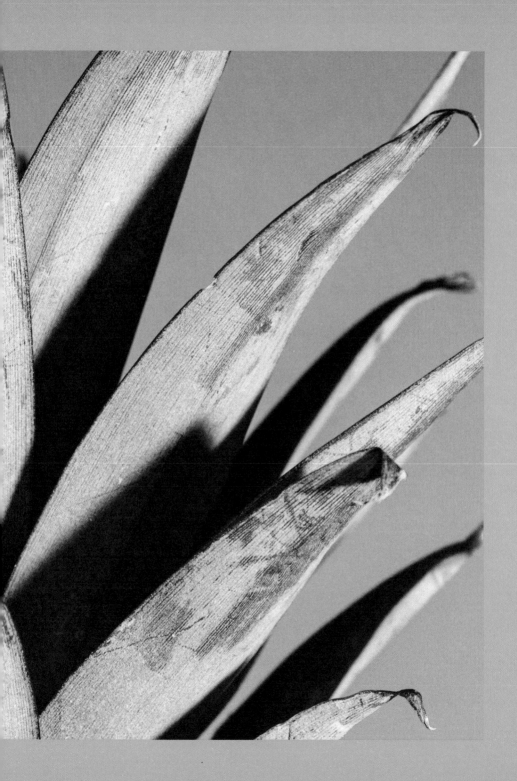

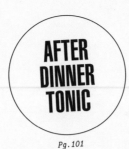

AFTER
DINNER
TONIC

Pg.101

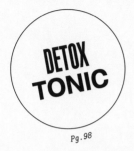

DETOX
TONIC

Pg.98

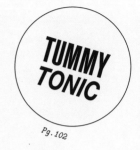

TUMMY
TONIC

Pg.102

Chapter 4

BLOATED?

IMPROVE DIGESTION.

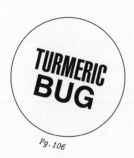

TURMERIC
BUG

Pg.106

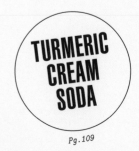

TURMERIC
CREAM
SODA

Pg.109

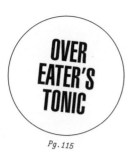

OVER EATER'S TONIC

Pg.115

Being bloated is a symptom of an unhappy digestive system. In order to banish the bloat, we need to improve the system. This chapter is all about toning the digestive system as a 'whole', using preventative tonics that support its various functions, in order to keep the bloat at bay.

We have to go further than seeing our guts just as plumbing. Health starts in the gut. It protects us from toxins, allergens, and infections. 70 per cent of the immune system sits inside it. It manages tens of trillions of bacteria in our colon, and maintains one of the most complex ecosystems on this planet. Drinking natural probiotics to regain healthy, balanced gut flora is essential in maintaining digestive health. So, learn to make your own, in the comfort of your home.

These tonics come in a range of forms: some are carminative herbal brews, others are fermented, fizzy and tangy; others are practically just vinegar. So really there's something for everyone here.

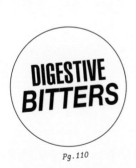

DIGESTIVE BITTERS

Pg.110

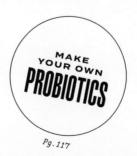

MAKE YOUR OWN PROBIOTICS

Pg.117

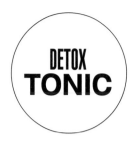

DETOX TONIC

A simple, soothing recipe with ancient Ayurverdic roots and heaps of benefits. CCF tea is brilliant for detoxification, digestion, and reducing bloating and gas. It stimulates the metabolism and clears out excess water retention.

This flushing action simultaneously cleanses the urinary tract and reduces inflammation. The mildly bitter carminative seeds rev up the detoxification process, purify the blood, and help to soothe a tense mind.

Ayurveda literally means 'the knowledge and wisdom of life'. It is a traditional system of holistic healing that originated in India over 5,000 years ago. Drinking artfully formulated Ayurvedic teas is a really effective way to reap the medicinal benefits of herbs and spices.

Cumin, coriander and fennel tea.

INGREDIENTS

Makes 2 servings
Ready in 8 minutes

500 ml (17 fl oz) water

¼ tsp cumin seeds

¼ tsp coriander seeds

¼ tsp fennel seeds

METHOD

Set the water to boil.

Meanwhile, toast the seeds in a dry frying pan (skillet), over a medium heat, until they become aromatic. Transfer the seeds to a pestle and mortar and bruise slightly.

Let the seeds steep in the boiled water for 5 minutes, or until it cools to a comfortable drinking temperature.

Strain out the spices and serve.

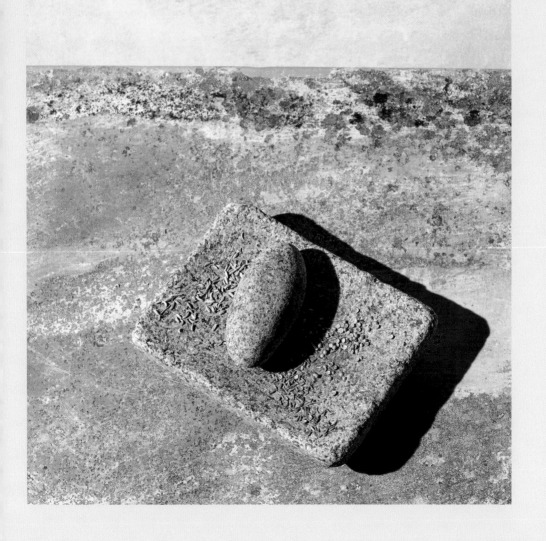

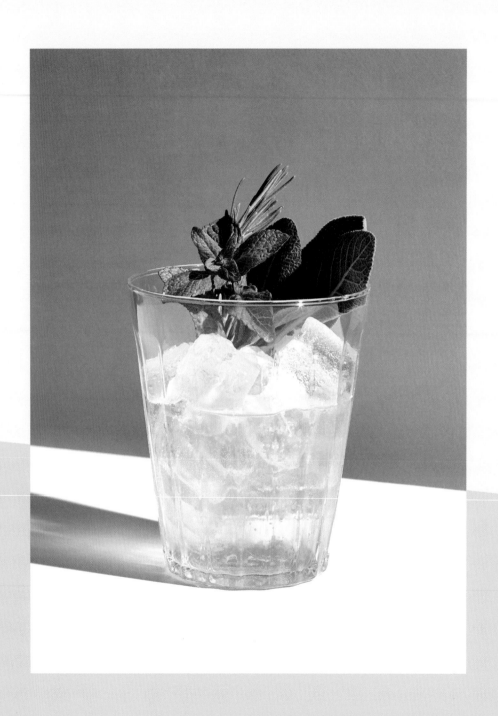

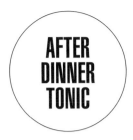

AFTER DINNER TONIC

A kombucha infused with ginger and a variety of herbs, such as rosemary, sage and mint, is the perfect tonic to sip on if you're feeling stuffed and bloated after a rather large meal.

A concoction of fresh herbs and bitters encourages the body to rev up the production of the digestive juices we need post-meal. Fresh ginger helps settle any queasiness as well.

Herbal kombucha with ginger.

INGREDIENTS

2.5-cm (1-in) piece of fresh ginger root

3 sage leaves

1 sprig of mint

1 sprig of rosemary

300 ml (10½ fl oz) shop-bought kombucha or Homemade Kombucha (see p. 118)

1–2 tsp digestive bitters (see p. 110)

QUICK METHOD

Makes 1 serving / Ready in 5 minutes

In a pestle and mortar, bash the ginger into a paste. Scoop into a glass, muddle with the fresh herbs. Stir in the kombucha and bitters. Strain and enjoy.

HOMEBREW METHOD

Makes 1 x 2 litre (70 fl oz) bottle /
Ready in 2–3 weeks

See p. 118. Once your kombucha is ready for its second fermentation, use the ingredients above to flavour it. Slice the ginger and bruise the herbs slightly. Put these into a sealable glass bottle of choice and fill to the top with the kombucha you have been brewing. Leave to brew for 2–3 weeks, or, if infusing into kombucha that's already made, just leave to stand in the fridge for 1 hour.

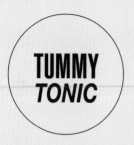

TUMMY TONIC

Ginger and tamarind are highly effective when it comes to upset stomachs. They have antifungal and antibacterial properties that help soothe discomfort and indigestion. They also have a calm and cooling effect on the intestinal tract.

Tamarind is one of the most widely used condiments in South-Asian kitchens. It's even in Worcestershire sauce and HP sauce. In traditional medicine, the pulp of the fruit, seeds, leaves, flowers and the bark are all used.

INGREDIENTS

Makes 350 ml
(12 fl oz) syrup
Ready in 40 minutes

200 ml (7 fl oz) water

100 g (3½ oz) fresh ginger root, thinly sliced or grated

200 g (7 oz/1 cup) coconut blossom nectar

METHOD FOR THE SPICY GINGER SYRUP

Bring the water, ginger and coconut blossom nectar to a simmer in a small saucepan over a medium heat, stirring, until the nectar has dissolved. Then gently simmer, uncovered, for about 30 minutes to reduce to syrup.

Strain the syrup through a fine mesh sieve. Leave to cool to room temperature. You can store it for up to 2 weeks, in sterilised bottles (see p. 19) in the fridge.

A refreshingly zingy ginger and tamarind cooler from tropical Thailand.

INGREDIENTS

Makes 6 servings
Ready in 30 minutes

200 g (7 oz) pliable block
of tamarind

1½ litres (52 fl oz)
filtered water

350 ml (12 fl oz) spicy
ginger syrup (see left)

pinch of sea salt

ice, to serve

1 litre (35 fl oz)
sparkling water, chilled

METHOD FOR THE COOLER

Break up the tamarind block with your fingers into a small heavy-based saucepan. Add 500 ml (17 fl oz) of the filtered water and bring up to a simmer, over a medium heat, stirring occasionally and breaking up the tamarind as it softens, about 20 minutes. Remove from the heat and let it stand for 15 minutes.

Strain the tamarind purée through a sieve into a bowl, pressing firmly to get all the flavour out. Discard the leftover pulp.

Whisk the tamarind purée, ginger syrup, remaining 1 litre (35 fl oz) of filtered water and salt together in a large jug (pitcher). Chill in the fridge until cold.

Once ready to drink, give the mixture a good stir, then pour into glasses filled two-thirds of the way with ice. Top off with sparkling water.

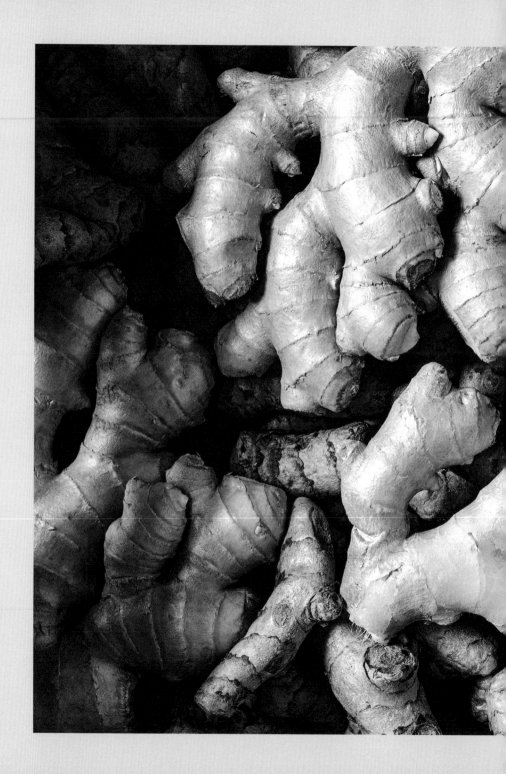

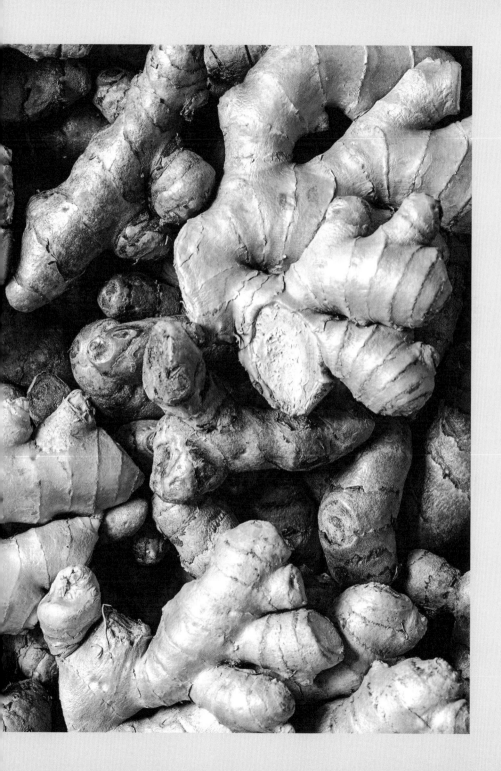

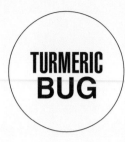

TURMERIC BUG

A 'bug' is a culture of beneficial bacteria, made from fresh ginger root and sugar. It is similar to a sourdough starter for bread or a SCOBY for making kombucha. Though not overly tasty by itself, the bug acts as the base for homemade tonics such as root beer, ginger beer and fruit 'sodas'. To make an authentic fermented soda, you need a bug.

The turmeric imparts its flavour and, as it naturally ferments, creates a mixture of beneficial bacteria. Rinse but don't peel the turmeric – the peel is rich in bacteria and yeast – and organic is best.

A homemade soda 'starter'.

INGREDIENTS

Makes 200 ml (7 fl oz)
Ready in approx.
3–5 days

200 g (7 oz) piece of fresh turmeric root, unpeeled

3–5 tbsp rapadura sugar or raw cane sugar

filtered water

METHOD

Chop the unpeeled turmeric root up finely or mash in a pestle and mortar. Transfer to a container with the lid left slightly ajar and keep on your kitchen counter.

Take 1 tablespoon of the turmeric paste and add to a glass jar with 1 tablespoon of the sugar and 3 tablespoons of filtered water. Mix well, cover, and place in a warm spot, around 22°C (72°F) is ideal.

Every day, add 1 tablespoon of turmeric paste, 1 tablespoon of sugar and 3 tablespoons of filtered water to the mixture, mix well, and leave to stand again.

Repeat until the turmeric bug is nice and bubbly. It can take between 3–5 days. Now you are ready to make Turmeric Cream Soda (see p. 108).

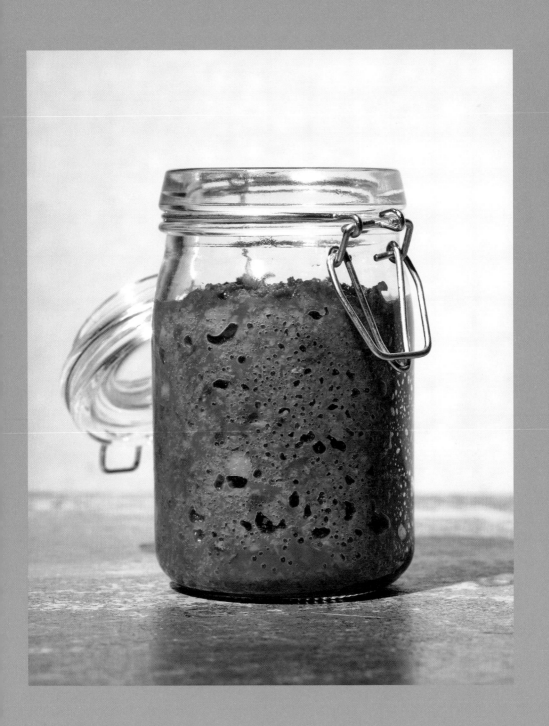

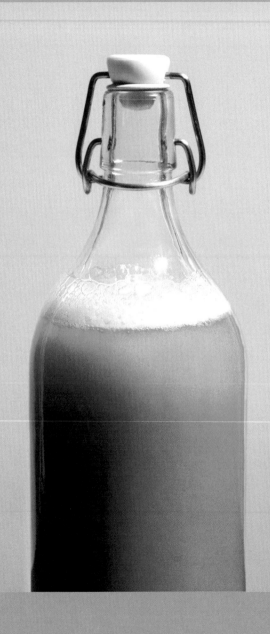

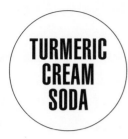

TURMERIC CREAM SODA

You deserve a treat, and this lightly sparkling, naturally fermented tonic is just that. The vanilla and lime give it an irresistible flavour and it's loaded with homemade probiotics too.

Our bodies struggle to absorb the benefits of raw turmeric. Fermenting the root to make soda is just another way to make it more bioavailable, and harvest valuable bacteria while you're at it. I make it the traditional way – no carbonators – just yeast, bacteria and sugar.

Fizzy turmeric, lime and vanilla tonic.

INGREDIENTS

Makes 2 litres (70 fl oz) Ready in approx. 5 days

750 ml (26 fl oz) filtered water, plus about 800–900 ml (28–32 fl oz) to top up

½ a vanilla pod

2.5-cm (1-inch) piece of fresh turmeric root, sliced

1 tsp crushed black peppercorns

170 ml (5½ fl oz) Turmeric Bug (see p. 106)

170 ml (5½ fl oz) fresh lime juice

50 g (1¾ oz/¼ cup) rapadura or raw cane sugar

Turmeric Beer Make a slightly alcoholic version by doubling the sugar.

METHOD

Once you have at least 170 ml (5½ fl oz) or more of bubbling Turmeric Bug starter, then you can start to make your soda tonic.

First, make turmeric tea. Fill a small saucepan with the 750 ml (26 fl oz) filtered water; add the vanilla, turmeric and pepper. Bring to the boil and then reduce the heat to simmer for 10 minutes. This process extracts as much flavour from the ingredients as possible.

Allow the tea to cool completely, and pour it (without straining) into your sterilised mason (preserving) jar (see p. 19). The boiled ingredients will continue to infuse. Stir in the turmeric bug, lime juice and sugar. Then top up the rest of the mason jar with filtered water, leaving about 5 cm (2 inches) of head room at the top.

Cover with a cloth and rubber band and leave in a shady spot away from direct sunlight. Allow it to ferment for around 3 days. It should taste sweet and sour when ready.

Now strain and pour into sterilised swing-top bottles (see p. 19). Leave the filled bottles in a shady spot, and let the natural yeasts get to work. Yeast releases CO_2 gasses that will make your soda fizzy. An overly hot room will accelerate the fermentation process, so it's worth putting your bottles into a cardboard box to contain potential explosions.

Check bottles daily for build up of fizz. Once they are fizzy (this should take 2 days), place them in the fridge, as they're ready to drink.

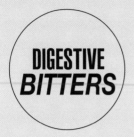

DIGESTIVE *BITTERS*

This is a tincture of bitter herbs, spices, roots and peels, infused in apple cider vinegar.

Bitter flavours get our digestive juices flowing. They help to soothe gas, burping, bloating and indigestion. They also balance our cravings for sweetness and keep our appetites in check, to prevent us from overindulging.

Sometime around 1824, Johann Siegert, a doctor in Venezuela, began making Angostura bitters as a stimulant for the troops, to help keep them on their feet. Even the ancient Egyptians were said to have infused medicinal herbs in jars of wine. Across Europe, bitters have been a core part of every meal, to prepare the digestive system for particularly heavy, fatty foods.

(Continues overleaf.)

INGREDIENTS

Makes as much as you like
Ready in 3 days

Note: all quantities depend on the size of your preserving jar.

(It's a good opportunity to use up what might be going to waste in your kitchen – choose from the list below.)

50% bitter-flavoured ingredients

50% aromatic ingredients

apple cider vinegar (enough to fill preserving jar)

METHOD

Chop your chosen ingredients up, or coarsely grind or crack them, to expose more surface area for infusion. Chuck it all into the large, sterilised glass jar.

Top up with apple cider vinegar, then seal, shake, and store at room temperature for 3 weeks.

Strain with a muslin (cheesecloth), then decant back into sterilised bottles and enjoy. It will keep for 3 months.

*For so much more
than a good cocktail
why not add a splash
of bitters?*

EQUIPMENT

large glass preserving jar
with lid, sterilised (see p. 19)

bottles for storage,
sterilised

muslin (cheesecloth)

BITTERS

Citrus peels: lemon, lime,
orange, grapefruit

Roots: liquorice root,
dandelion root, turmeric
root, ginger root

AROMATICS

Spices: allspice, aniseed
(anise), caraway, cardamom,
celery seed, chillies,
cinnamon, cloves, coriander
seeds, fennel, ground ginger,
juniper berries, nutmeg,
peppercorns, star anise,
vanilla pods

Herbs and flowers:
chamomile, hibiscus, hops,
lavender, lemongrass, mint,
rose, rosemary, sage, thyme

Nuts: toasted almonds,
pecans, walnuts

Beans: cacao beans, cocoa
nibs, coffee beans

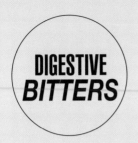

DIGESTIVE
BITTERS

NOTES

Keep this tincture on your kitchen counter and splash a drop or two into any drink, to give it an extra dimension and tonic-like quality.

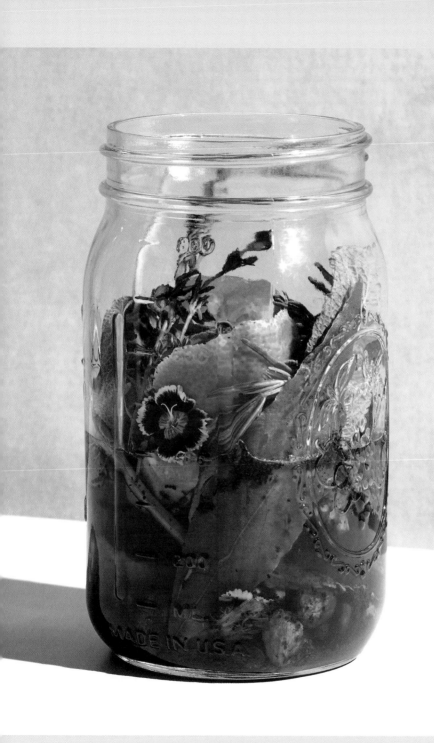

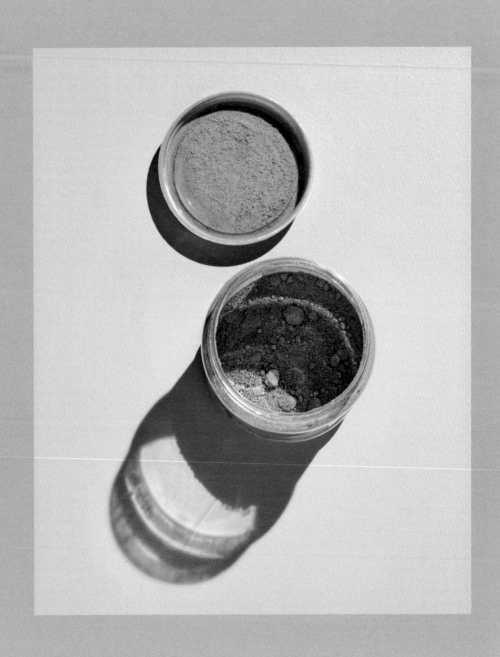

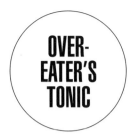

OVER-EATER'S TONIC

A digestive tonic inspired by a colourful Indian post-supper snack called *mukhwas* that I discovered at a restaurant situated in the car park of a very sacred Hindu temple near Wembley, London. Not only did the menu adhere entirely to the Hindu practice of Sattvic eating (a vegetarian diet of unprocessed, healing foods), but it was also some of the tastiest Indian food I have ever eaten. *Mukhwas* is mostly made using fennel seeds, peppermint oil, sesame seeds, coconut and sugar. Chewing *mukhwas* (fennel seeds in particular) after meals, to support digestion, is an age-old tradition in India and Pakistan.

Fennel and peppermint jump-start the digestive process, by encouraging the production of digestive juices, and also destroy the bacteria that cause bad breath (halitosis), making them brilliant mouth fresheners as well.

INGREDIENTS

Makes 1 serving
Ready in 5 minutes

1 tsp fennel seeds

1 tbsp honey

2.5-cm (1-inch) piece of fresh ginger root

2.5-cm (1-inch) piece of fresh turmeric root or ¼ tsp turmeric powder

1 sprig of peppermint

juice of 1 orange

juice of 1 lime

240 ml (8 fl oz) sparkling water

1 tbsp apple cider vinegar

METHOD

In a frying pan (skillet) set over a medium heat, dry-toast the fennel seeds.

Transfer the seeds to a pestle and mortar, and mash with the honey, ginger, turmeric and peppermint, to release their essential oils. This will create the base of your drink.

Transfer this mixture to a glass and stir in the remaining ingredients, until mixed. Add the digestive bitters (if using), strain and serve over ice.

OPTIONAL *1-2 teaspoons Digestive Bitters (see p. 110)*

After-dinner fennel, turmeric and orange spritzer.

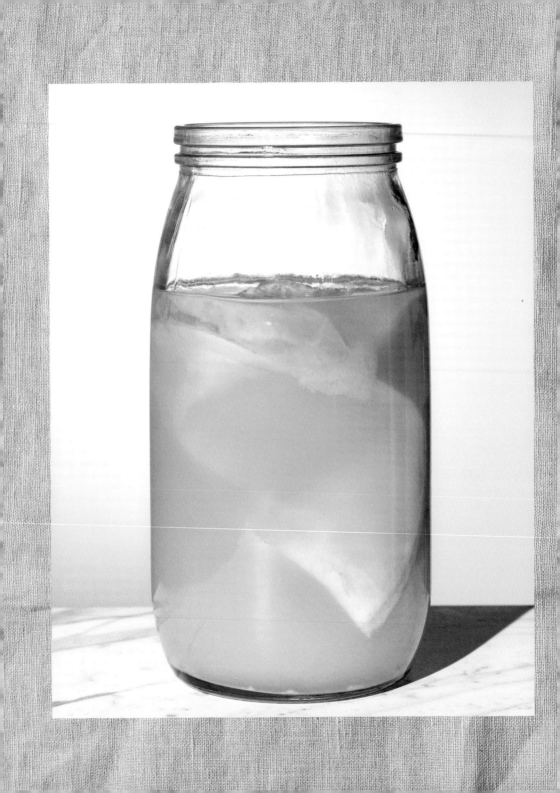

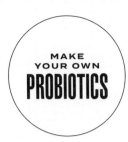

MAKE YOUR OWN PROBIOTICS

My friend Bertel is the kombucha king. He's also the most relaxed, Birkenstock-wearing, unassuming dude I know. Here's his recipe – so easy and so forgiving, if you're busy, lazy or both.

Simply put, kombucha is a fermented tea. Fermenting tea and sugar with a starter culture is how you make it. The taste is surprisingly delicious, something between sparkling apple cider and Champagne – it all depends on the type of tea you use.

The fermentation process creates essential acids that help to detoxify the body, regulate the blood's pH level, and which are a source of natural antibiotics, that keep both the immune and digestive systems healthy. Kombucha provides a source of probiotic micro-organisms that are very beneficial to the health of our guts.

Since it's naturally fermented with a living colony of bacteria and yeast, this has a myriad of beneficial effects, such as improving digestion, fighting candida (harmful yeast) overgrowth, and stabilising mood.

The first recorded use of kombucha comes from China in 221 BC, during the Tsin Dynasty. It was known as 'the tea of immortality'. It has also been used in Eastern Europe, Russia and Japan for several centuries.

(Recipe continued overleaf.)

Homemade kombucha by Bertel Haugen.

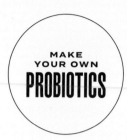

**MAKE
YOUR OWN
PROBIOTICS**

INGREDIENTS

a SCOBY (Symbiotic Colony
of Bacteria and Yeast) –
also known as a 'mother'
or 'mushroom'. You can buy
these online, or ask a friend
that is already brewing
kombucha at home.

4 green, white, oolong
or black tea bags

3 heaped tbsp raw cane
sugar

EQUIPMENT

a 5-litre (5-quart) glass
vessel with a tap or spigot
on the bottom

a 2-litre (70 fl oz) glass jar
for brewing tea

close-weave muslin cloths
(cheesecloths)

elastic bands

glass bottles for storage
(swing-top/stoppered
preserving bottles are
the best – they need to
be completely airtight.
See p. 19)

a funnel

a small sieve

METHOD

Clean all equipment thoroughly with boiling water rather than soap.
SCOBYs don't like soap.

Put your SCOBY into your 5-litre (5-quart) brewing vessel.

Put the green tea bags into the 2-litre (70-fl oz) jar, along with
the sugar and fill about ¼ of the jar with boiling water. Stir until the
sugar dissolves to create your sweet tea concentrate.

Let the tea brew for 10 minutes, then remove the tea bags from
the jar.

Top up the jar with fresh filtered cold water – this way you dilute
the sweet tea concentrate and cool it down quicker.

Wait until the brewed tea is lukewarm, then pour it into your
brewing jar on top of the SCOBY. Mix gently with a wooden spoon.
Don't worry if the SCOBY sinks, breaks or anything really – it is fine.

Cover the brewing vessel with the cloth and elastic band.
It needs to breathe, but you don't want flies or anything else
getting in there.

Take a small amount of liquid out via the tap to taste it. It should
taste like sweet green tea. Now, sit back, relax, and let the SCOBY
do its work. The SCOBY will get to work on your sweet tea. It will
digest the sugar and tea to make kombucha. It will also form a new
SCOBY on the top of the jar. This might start to look quite weird and
misshapen, but it's fine. It's incredibly robust and the acidity of the
kombucha liquid will make sure that nothing nasty can get in. If you
see any mould developing on the SCOBY then something has gone
wrong. Throw all the liquid and SCOBYs away if this happens and
start again.

After a week, take some liquid out of the jar, via the tap, and taste
it. If it tastes too sweet, then you need to wait longer. If it tastes
sour and fermented, then you are ready for part two; flavouring it.

FLAVOURING YOUR BOOCH

First, sterilise your bottles with boiling water (see p. 19).

Mash or chop up your fruit, spices and flavourings of choice into a paste or into small enough pieces that will easily fit in the bottles (see p. 120).

Fill each bottle about 2–3 cm (1 inch) deep with your chopped up fruit and flavourings. There are no rules here, just go with your gut.

Remove the muslin cloth from your brewing vessel. Stir the liquid with a wooden spoon. Don't worry about breaking the SCOBYs (by now there should be two in there). Mixing up the liquid will help ensure that the yeasts are evenly distributed, which will help build fizzy kombucha.

Using your funnel, fill the bottles up with kombucha liquid from the brewing vessel. Fill it up right to the top of the bottle – you want as little air as possible in there. This also helps with fizziness. Seal the bottles and make sure they're airtight.

Note: you can take out as much kombucha as you want from the brewing vessel, but you need to leave enough in there for the SCOBY to thrive. I tend to take out 2 litres (70 fl oz) at a time.
You can then refill the vessel with 2 litres (70 fl oz) of sweet tea, so starting the process again.

You should now have 2–3 bottles filled with fruit and kombucha, all nicely sealed and looking great. Leave them out at room temperature to ferment. The second fermentation in the bottle is anaerobic, meaning that carbon dioxide will build up and eventually become fizzy. The kombucha will also extract any colour from the fruit inside.

Wait at least a week before you test your bottles for fizz. Only try one, and if it isn't fizzy, then wait a few more days. It can take 2–3 weeks sometimes to get fizzy kombucha, so have patience.

Once the kombucha is fizzy, it's ready to serve. Put 1 bottle in the fridge. Serve chilled, and sieve before serving, to keep out any pieces of fruit or spice.

As long as your SCOBY is healthy, it is content to sit in the kombucha liquid for weeks on end. You don't need to 'feed' it like a sourdough culture. Just bear in mind that, the longer you leave it, the more sour it gets. If it's too sour, take some liquid out and add more brewed chilled sweet tea.

Be patient and wait for the fizz!

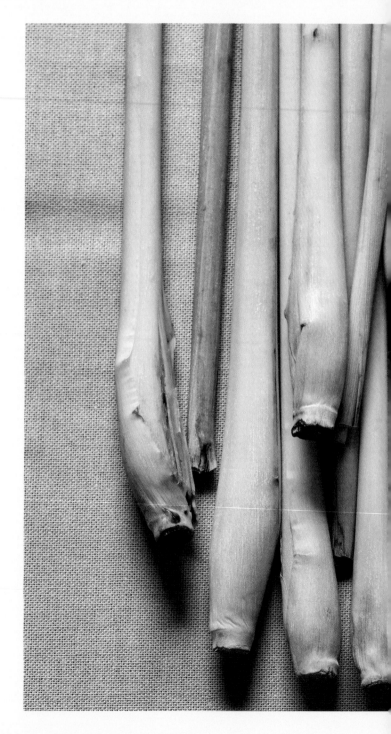

DELICIOUS INGREDIENTS FOR YOUR KOMBUCHA

Fruit:
raspberries,
strawberries, kiwis,
oranges, clementines,
pomegranates,
wild blackberries,
blueberries,
pineapple, mango,
peaches, apricots,
apples, pears, etc.

Fresh spices:
fresh ginger is
amazing! Fresh
turmeric is also
really great - it
adds an earthy
flavour and amazing
colour to your
kombucha

Dried spices:
cinnamon, cloves,
nutmeg, vanilla,
star anise, coriander
seeds, etc.

Fresh / dried herbs:
rosemary, lavender,
thyme, mint,
lemon balm

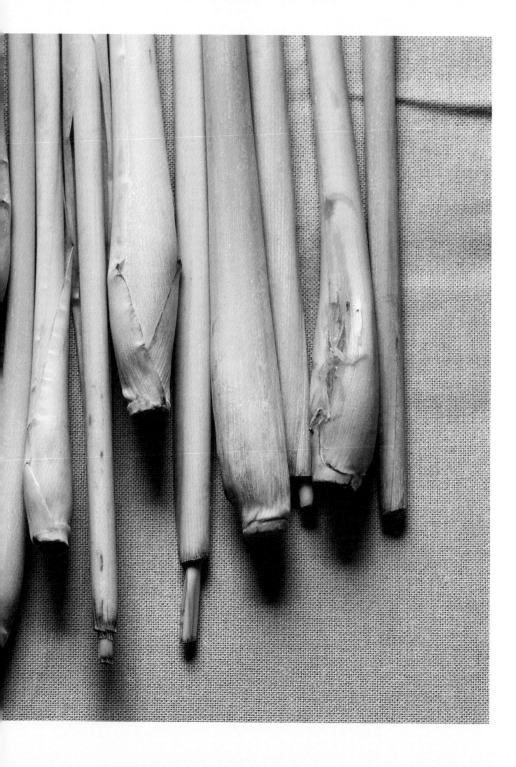

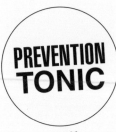

PREVENTION TONIC

Pg. 126

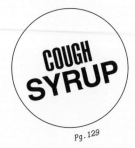

COUGH SYRUP

Pg. 129

FEVER GRASS TONIC

Pg. 125

Chapter 5

SICK?

RAMP UP THE IMMUNE SYSTEM TO FIGHT THE COLD THE NATURAL WAY: WITH HERBS, SPICES, PLENTY OF SLEEP, FLUIDS AND THE LIKE. MAKE A TONIC.

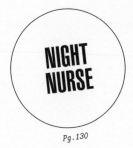

NIGHT NURSE

Pg. 130

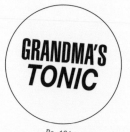

GRANDMA'S TONIC

Pg. 134

A chapter for times of need when colds and flu ravage the body, you're stuffed with phlegm, and riddled with aches and pains.

These tonics replenish the body and soothe symptoms with potent anti-inflammatory powers, and boost the immune system to prevent the symptoms from coming back.

So, with that in mind, it's time to jump off the complaint train, drag yourself over to your kitchen cupboard, and get on with the healing.

Here's a run-down of cold and flu treatments that don't require a trip to the pharmacy, but are good for you, and somehow taste good too.

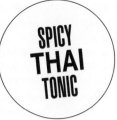

Pg. 135

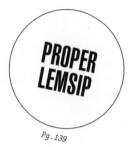

Pg. 139

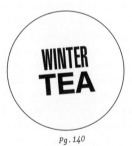

Pg. 140

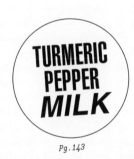

Pg. 143

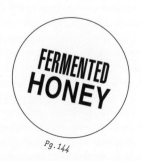

Pg. 144

* Since 70 per cent of the immune system sits in the gut, I'd recommend checking out the Bloated chapter after this one, for extra preventative measures (see p. 96).

** Stress and anxiety have a negative impact on your immune system – there's a chapter for that too (see p. 46).

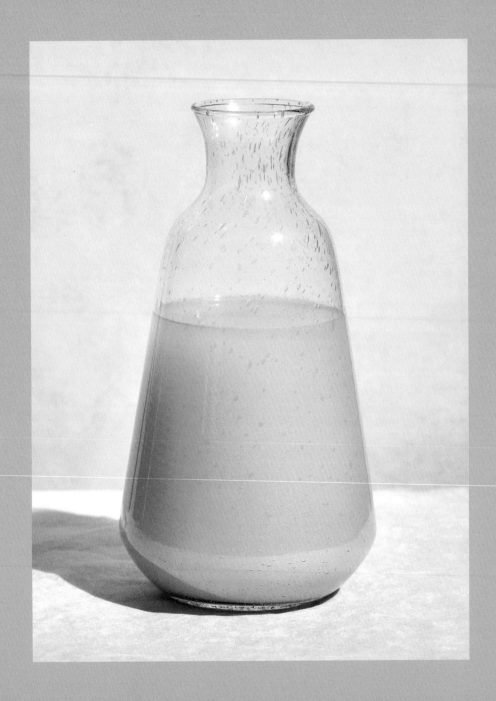

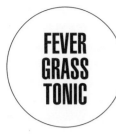

FEVER GRASS TONIC

A tart and thirst-quenching blend of apple cider vinegar, honey, and water infused with zingy ginger- and lemongrass flavours, to help you cope with the nasty symptoms of cold and flu.

This recipe is based on the 'Switchel', which is derived from 'Oxymel', an ancient Greek medicinal tonic made from vinegar, honey and water.

Lemongrass has antibacterial and antifungal properties and is packed with vitamin C that boosts your immune system in order to fight infections. It's the reason Jamaicans call it 'fever grass'.

Ginger is also a powerful painkiller. Consuming small amounts of it can be as effective at reducing symptoms of pain and inflammation as over-the-counter painkillers. So, next time you feel a headache coming on, switchel it up.

INGREDIENTS

Makes about 2 litres
(70 fl oz)
Ready in 40 minutes

2 cloves

½ a cinnamon stick

2 litres (70 fl oz) filtered water

200 g (7 oz) fresh ginger root, unpeeled, rinsed and sliced into chunks

3 lemongrass stalks, finely sliced

juice of 2 lemons

apple cider vinegar, to taste

honey, to taste

METHOD

In a medium, heavy-based saucepan over a medium heat, dry toast the spices, until they become aromatic. Crumble the cinnamon slightly, and then add the water to the pan, letting it all infuse over a low–medium heat for 15 minutes.

In the meantime, add the chunks of ginger and lemongrass slices to a blender, and blend with a little bit of water to create a fine paste.

Once the water and spices have infused, turn off the heat, and add the ginger and lemongrass paste to the mixture. Add the lemon juice, stir well, and let the concoction cool to room temperature.

When cool, add the vinegar and honey to taste. Store in the fridge for up to 20 days.

Nature's paracetamol.

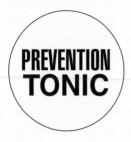

PREVENTION TONIC

Time to take all preventative health measures possible. Even if you eat fermented foods all the time, a little extra protection can't hurt. This tonic pickles the most potent of roots and spices to create a fiery liquid supplement that will tackle any signs of weakness. Drink a tablespoon with a glass of water every morning.

The ingredients are simple, and loaded with good things that each have health-enhancing properties. Once fermented, they become more digestible, and packed with healthy immunity-boosting bacteria.

Because winter is coming

INGREDIENTS

Makes 8 servings
Ready in 3 weeks

8 cm (3 in) piece of fresh turmeric root, unpeeled

18 cm (7 in) piece of fresh ginger root, unpeeled

200 g (7 oz) red bird's eye chillies (Thai chillies) or habaneros, without stems

3 bulbs garlic, peeled

3 white onions, peeled

pinch of sea salt

1 litre (35 fl oz) filtered water

EQUIPMENT

a 2-litre (70-fl oz) glass vessel

muslin (cheesecloth) and an elastic band

METHOD

Rinse your turmeric, ginger, chillies and horseradish (if using) thoroughly. Leave the skins on.

Slice all of the ingredients into thin disks. I like to use a mandolin – this way you can layer evenly, and the ingredients become beautiful edible pickles once ready. You can slice the chillies in half.

Place the turmeric, garlic and ginger slices in the bottom of your vessel, top with the chillies, then with the onions, then with herbs and lemon slices (if using), finally placing the horseradish slices across the top so as to form an almost flat layer.

Mix salt into the filtered water and then slowly pour it over the veggie layers until they are submerged. Cover the vessel with the cloth and secure with an elastic band.

Allow the mixture to ferment at room temperature for 3 weeks. After this time, strain the liquid and bottle it into sterilised bottles (see p. 19). You can eat the pickles at this point too.

Store in the fridge until ready to serve. It will keep for up to 3 months.

OPTIONAL *200g (7 oz) horseradish root; unpeeled sprigs of rosemary; thyme or oregano or 1 lemon*

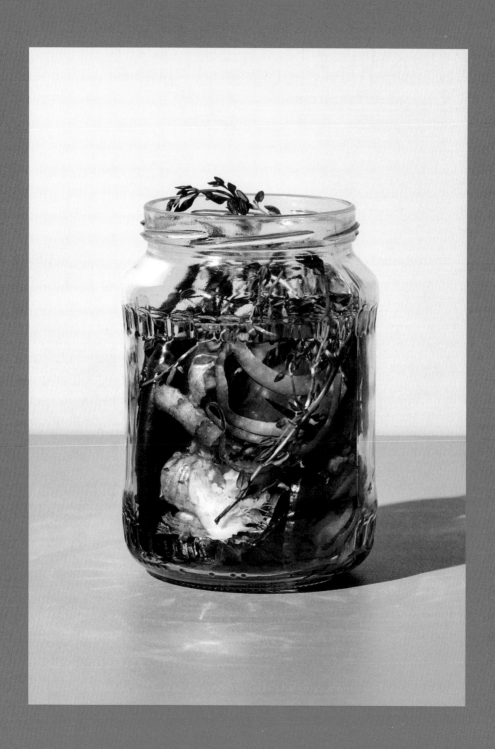

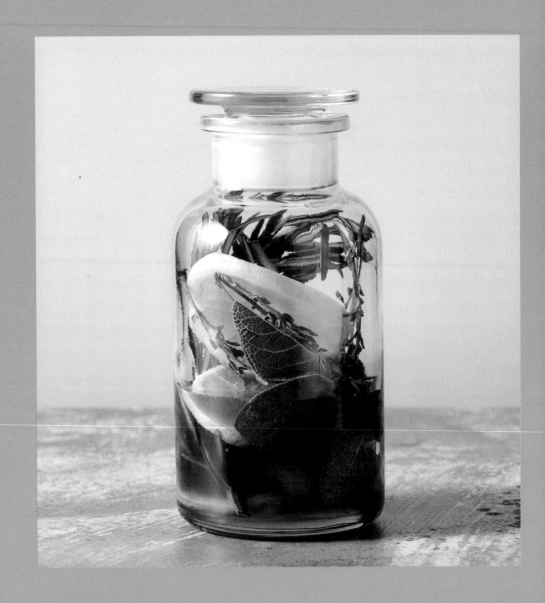

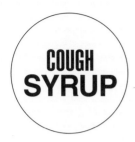

COUGH SYRUP

A DIY cough syrup made from kitchen cupboard staples, to help you combat your cough as well as reduce inflammation in the throat. Sip it by the tablespoon until your itchy, scratchy throat is content.

Honey and lemon is a legendary combination when it comes to sore throats. Combine that with anti-fungal herbs to open up the airways, and loosen up and expel mucus from the lungs.

You'll be winning in no time.

INGREDIENTS

Makes 360 ml
(12 fl oz)
Ready in 20 minutes

180 ml (6 fl oz)
extra-virgin olive oil

3 lemons, sliced

fresh sprigs of sage,
rosemary and thyme

180 ml (6 fl oz) honey
or Fermented Honey
(see p. 144)

METHOD

Add all the ingredients, except for the honey, to a small saucepan set over a medium heat. Infuse for 5 minutes, then remove from the heat and let it cool.

Once cool, strain, mix the honey in well, and store in a sterilised mason (preserving) jar (see p. 19) or other container with a tight-fitting lid.

It will keep in the fridge for 3 months, or keep on your kitchen counter for about 1½ months.

OPTIONAL *2½ cm (1 in) piece of fresh turmeric or ginger root, grated*

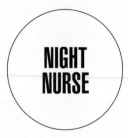

NIGHT NURSE

This herbal tea remedy combines comforting, sleep-inducing spices with a homemade cough syrup, to relieve tickly coughs and sore throats.

The medicinal pantry is full of sleep aids. Combining spices such as cinnamon and nutmeg creates a synergistic sedative effect on the body, that helps to restore calm. Honey also facilitates a good night's sleep, by stabilising blood sugar levels and contributing to the release of melatonin in the brain, a hormone responsible for inducing sleep.

Sleep like a baby.

INGREDIENTS

Makes 8 servings
Ready in 2-3 hours

3 cinnamon sticks

1 tbsp cloves

½ tsp black
peppercorns

15 bay leaves

¼ tsp grated nutmeg

5-cm (2-inch) piece of fresh
ginger root, finely sliced

2 litres (70 fl oz)
filtered water

1 tbsp DIY Cough
Syrup (see p. 129) or honey

METHOD

Combine all the ingredients together (except for the cough syrup and honey) in a large saucepan.

Bring to the boil, then reduce to a very low heat, and allow the ingredients to steep for 2–3 hours.

Strain, and serve with a tablespoon of DIY cough syrup or honey stirred into your mug. Feel free to add a dash of your milk of choice too, if you wish.

OPTIONAL *milk of your choice*

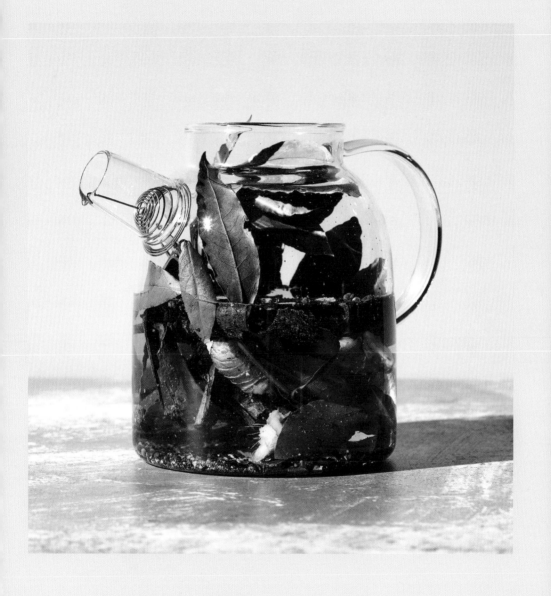

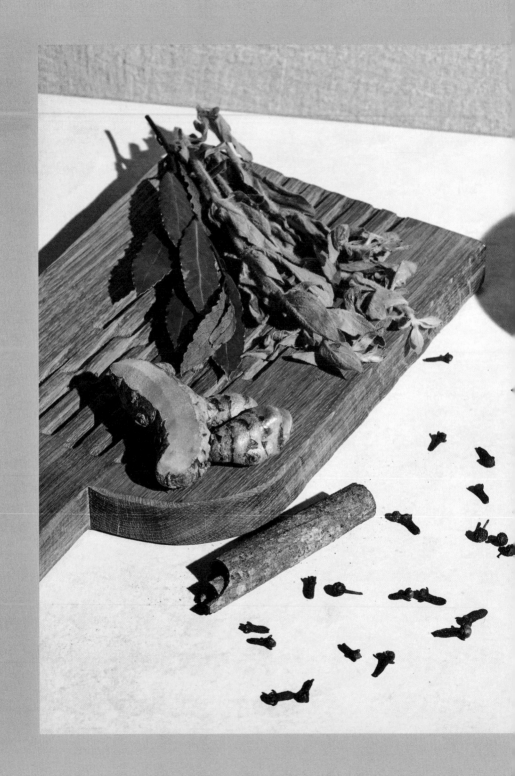

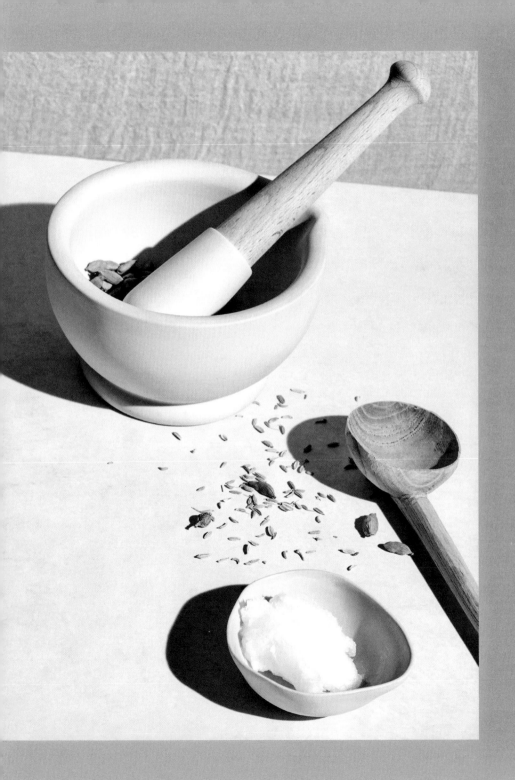

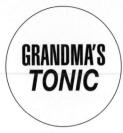

GRANDMA'S TONIC

Indian grandmas know a thing or two about colds. This is a traditional healing tea from India, known as *kadha*, made with humble kitchen healers.

This is an all-encompassing wellness tonic to get you feeling healthier and stronger in no time.

The earliest form of chai, didn't have any tea in it, but was rather a simple combination of plant roots, bark, seeds and spices. Legend has it that an Indian prince concocted the recipe in a quest to create a healing elixir. After that, the recipe was adapted according to the ancient practice of Ayurvedic holistic medicine.

To remedy a cold.

INGREDIENTS

Makes 4–5 cups
Ready in 10 minutes

2 cloves

crack of freshly ground black pepper

2 green cardamom pods

¼ tsp fennel seeds

1 litre (35 fl oz) filtered water

1 tsp grated fresh ginger root

5–6 leaves of holy basil or regular basil

½ tsp ghee or coconut oil

honey, to taste

METHOD

In a heavy-based saucepan, over a medium heat, dry roast the whole spices (cloves, pepper, cardamom, fennel, cinnamon and bay leaf, if using), until they become aromatic.

Pour in the water, add the ginger, turmeric (if using) and bring to the boil. You can also add the optional saffron at this stage.

Once boiling, turn down the heat, add the basil and simmer for 5 minutes.

Remove from the heat, strain and pour into a cup. Add ghee or coconut oil, and some honey to taste.

OPTIONAL *1 small cinnamon stick; 1 bay leaf; ½ tsp turmeric powder or 2½ cm (1 in) piece of grated fresh turmeric root; 2–3 strands of saffron*

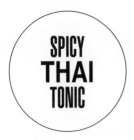

SPICY THAI TONIC

A hot and sour kombucha to crush your cold, packed with the flavours of Thailand's favourite cure-all soup, tom yum is light, cleansing and restorative.

Chilli and fresh citrus fruits are packed with vitamin C. Galangal and lemongrass really help clear the sinuses, and the probiotics within kombucha will do wonders for restoring your immune system.

Although early Thai home cooks weren't food scientists, their resourcefulness and creativity resulted in dishes packed with herbs and spices, with flavour and health benefits to match. Today, these benefits have been scientifically proven, suggesting that a daily spicy bowl of tom yum might help keep the doctor away.

INGREDIENTS

Makes as much as you like
Ready in 3 days

1 stalk lemongrass

2.5-cm (1-inch) piece of galangal root

½ a lime

1 kaffir lime leaf

½ a lemon

300 ml (10½ fl oz) store-bought kombucha or Homemade Kombucha (see p. 118)

½ chopped fresh red chilli, deseeded (optional)

QUICK METHOD

Makes 1 serving / Ready in 5 minutes

In a pestle and mortar, bruise the lemongrass and galangal. Add to a glass and muddle with the other ingredients and the chilli, if using. Strain and enjoy.

HOMEBREW METHOD

Makes a 2 litre (70 fl oz) bottle /
Ready in 2-3 weeks

See p. 118. Once your kombucha is ready for its second fermentation, use the ingredients left to flavour it. Crush the lemongrass, grate the galangal and bruise the herbs slightly, then put all the ingredients into a sealable sterilised glass bottle of choice (see p. 19) and fill to the top with the kombucha you have been brewing. Leave to brew for 2-3 weeks.

Tom yum kombucha.

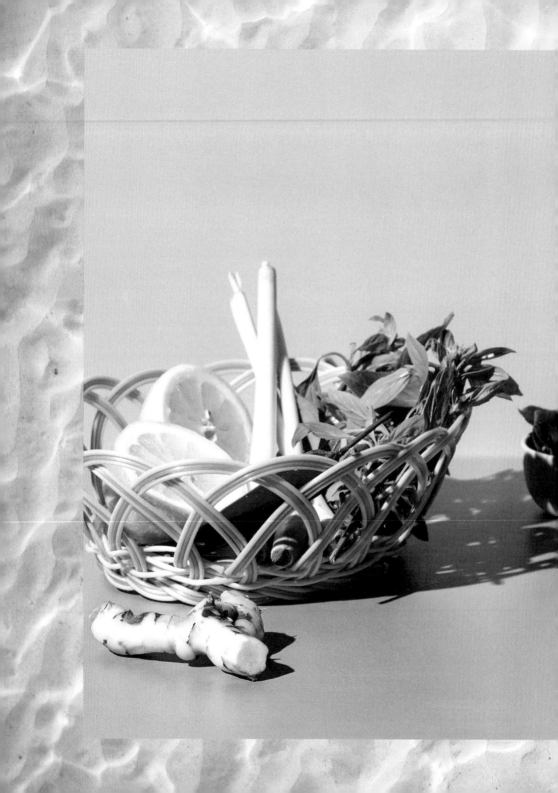

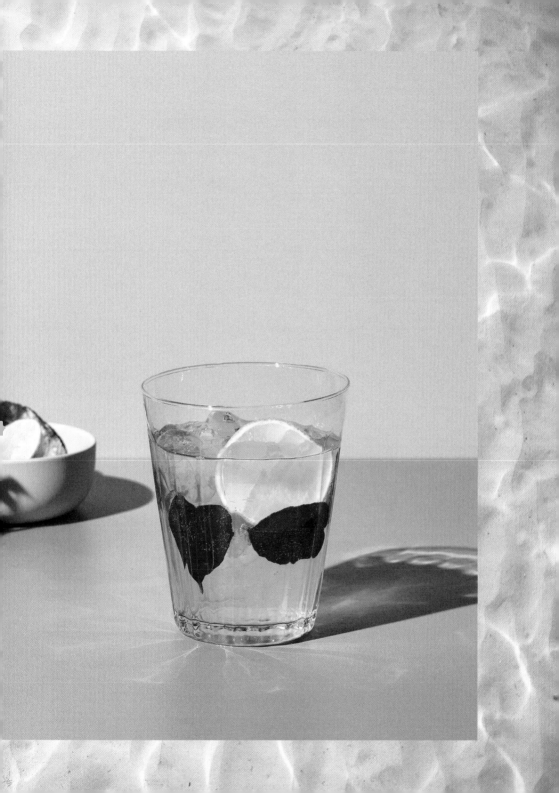

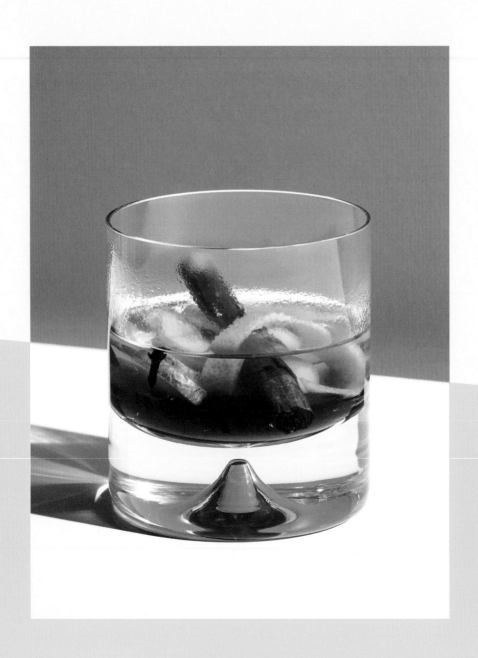

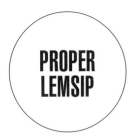

PROPER LEMSIP

A tonic to bring a glow to the chilled and fragile, by stoking the internal fire. Hot toddies were a staple saviour during the freezing cold days and nights I spent studying in Edinburgh, Scotland; there couldn't be a better drink to make you feel cosy.

Whisky is a great decongestant, and the booze helps you sleep. There is such a thing as too many hot toddies though – moderation is key, if your goal is to feel better. The heat, spice, sweet and sour flavours also encourage mucus production, to help you blow out any bacteria and viruses.

The name 'toddy' comes from Tod's Well, a spring on Arthur's Seat, which is a famous hill in the heart of Edinburgh. The Scots originally made toddies to make their whisky more palatable, but even after refining the distilling methods, they kept their fondness for this tonic, after realising that drinking it regularly both prevented and relieved colds.

INGREDIENTS

Makes 1 serving
Ready in 10 minutes

250 ml (9 fl oz)
just-boiled water

1 cinnamon stick

2 cloves

2.5-cm (1-inch) piece of
fresh ginger root, sliced

1 tbsp honey or
Fermented Honey
(see p. 144)

1 slice of lemon

2 tbsp whisky

METHOD

Add all the ingredients to a small teapot or glass and leave to brew for 5 minutes. Once infused, enjoy right away.

Hot toddy tonic.

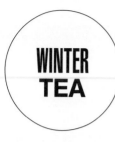

WINTER TEA

This is a quick recipe to have to hand when you suspect a cold is coming on, or you just want to warm up with a cosy drink after a long, dark and blustery day.

Herbal teas help to boost both our physical and mental health. Fresh herbs are high in antioxidants and help to decrease inflammation; they have great therapeutic virtues as well. A pinch of cayenne thins mucus, and can therefore clear up your nasal passages.

The first cup of herbal tea was born by accident thousands of years ago. Legend has it that, in 2737 BC, a Chinese Emperor named Shen-Nung was boiling some water to purify it, when some leaves from a nearby bush unexpectedly blew into the pot without his knowledge. Naturally, the brew became aromatic, so he became curious and tasted it, prompting him to spend the rest of his days tasting hundreds of varieties of herbs, to test their medicinal values.

A one-pot wonder

INGREDIENTS

Makes 1 cup
Ready in 10 minutes

300 ml (10½ fl oz) water

½ a lime

½ a lemon

3 cm (1¼ in) piece of fresh ginger root, sliced

pinch of cayenne pepper

1 sprig each fresh mint, thyme and rosemary

½ a cinnamon stick

honey, to taste

METHOD

Boil the water in a heavy-based saucepan.

Give your lemon and lime a good squeeze into the pan, then add them to the brew whole.

Now add the remainder of the ingredients (except for the honey) to the brew. Reduce the heat and simmer for 5 minutes.

Add honey to taste, then strain and serve.

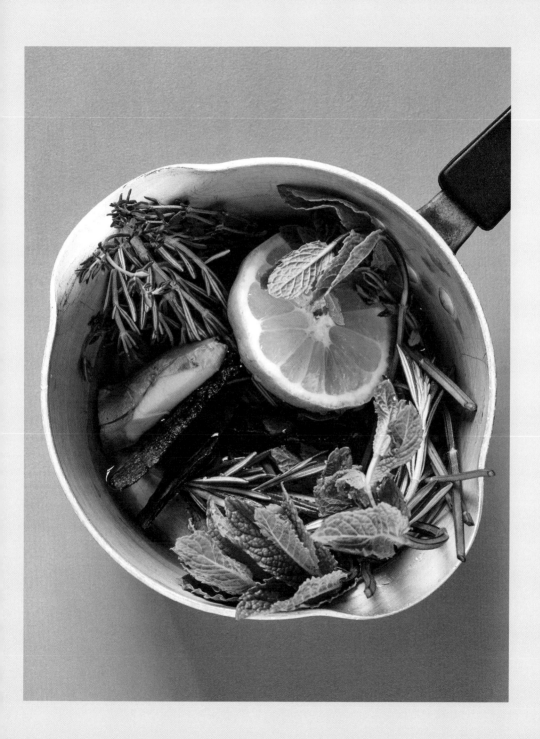

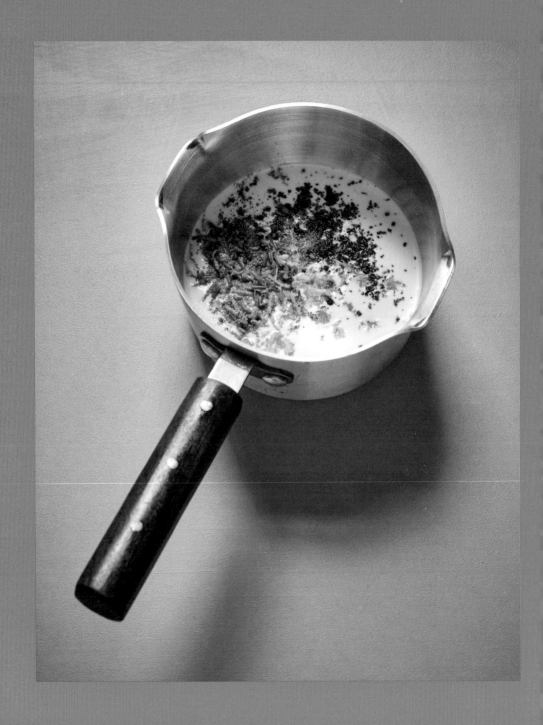

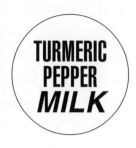

TURMERIC PEPPER *MILK*

Pepper milk is a creamy, age-old remedy, to keep the immune system strong and prevent illness. More commonly known as 'golden milk', this version is laced with black gold. Fresh turmeric and freshly ground black pepper sets this latte apart from the rest.

Black pepper increases the bioavailability of cumin, the essential compound of turmeric that is responsible for its anti-inflammatory, antioxidant, and antimicrobial properties. The pepper itself has potent anti-inflammatory, antioxidant, antibacterial, fever-reducing, and immune-boosting properties as well.

This 'latte' actually has a long, rich tradition that dates back thousands of years. Within the ancient system of medicine in India known as Ayurveda, turmeric pepper milk is a tonic that's meant to be nourishing, and delicious too.

If doctors could prescribe lattes, this would be it

INGREDIENTS

Makes 1 big cup
Ready in 10 minutes

1½ tsp black peppercorns

250 ml (9 fl oz) pure coconut milk

100 ml (3 fl oz) filtered water

1 tbsp grated fresh turmeric root or 1 tsp ground turmeric

1 tsp grated fresh ginger root

2 tsp coconut blossom nectar

pinch of sea salt

METHOD

In a frying pan (skillet) over a medium heat, dry-toast the black peppercorns until they become aromatic. Crush them in a black pepper grinder or a pestle and mortar.

In a small saucepan, bring the coconut milk and water to a light simmer, then add the turmeric, ginger, coconut blossom nectar and salt. Continue to simmer, stirring, for about 5 minutes, until well infused.

Filter the tonic through a fine mesh sieve. Add the crushed black pepper to the mixture and it's ready to serve.

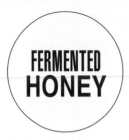

FERMENTED HONEY

Honey is antimicrobial and antibacterial – a total rock star for your immune system. It's great at soothing itchy/scratchy throats and at lasting indefinitely in your pantry. It's a staple. And yes, you can ferment it.

Honey has been used as food and medicine around the world for thousands of years. Hippocrates, an ancient Greek scientist, prescribed a simple diet, favouring honey taken as *oxymel* (vinegar and honey) for pain, *hydromel* (water and honey) for thirst, and a mixture of honey, water and various herbs for fevers.

The east of Turkey is famous for an old-world mystery; a dark; honey made from the pollen of the opium poppy, known as *Deli Bal* or 'mad honey'. The poppy, or rather opium, was highly valued by the ancient Greeks and Egyptians for its painkilling and sleep-inducing qualities. This nectar is fiery, mouth numbing and lightly hallucinogenic. Yet in Turkey, people consider it a type of medicine – a sleepy treat reserved for those in the know.

The treat of all treats.

INGREDIENTS

water (approx. 1 part water to 8 parts honey)

Raw, unpasteurised honey (the key is to find the minimally processed stuff – ideally with the crystallised crunchy bits of honeycomb still in it)

METHOD

Stir a small amount of water into the honey and leave the jar on the kitchen counter, with the lid resting on top but not fastened.

Give it a good stir every day.

After two weeks, the honey should start to bubble like a sourdough starter and smell sour. You should be left with a honey that's sweet and tangy with a thick, whipped marshmallow texture.

Use it to sweeten your tonics.

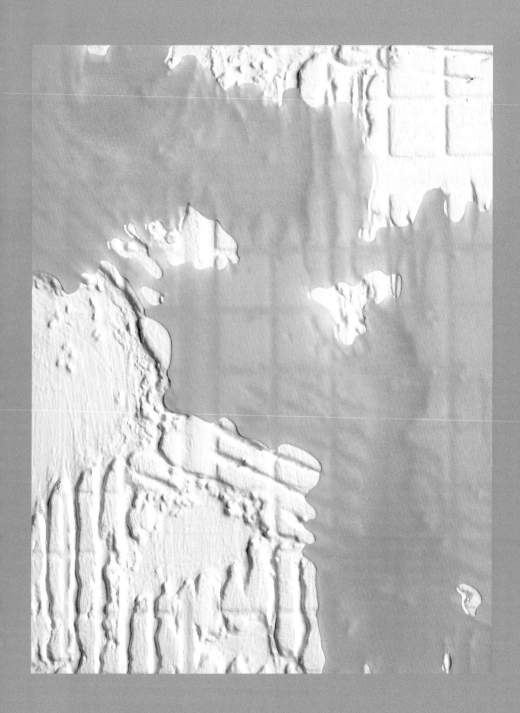

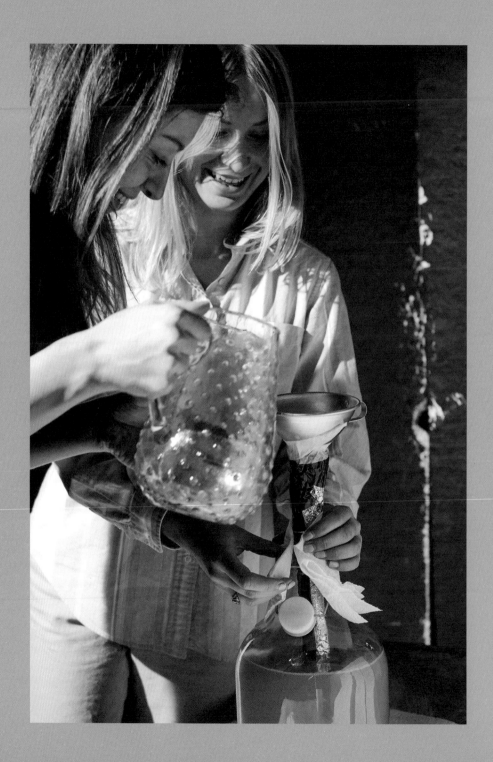

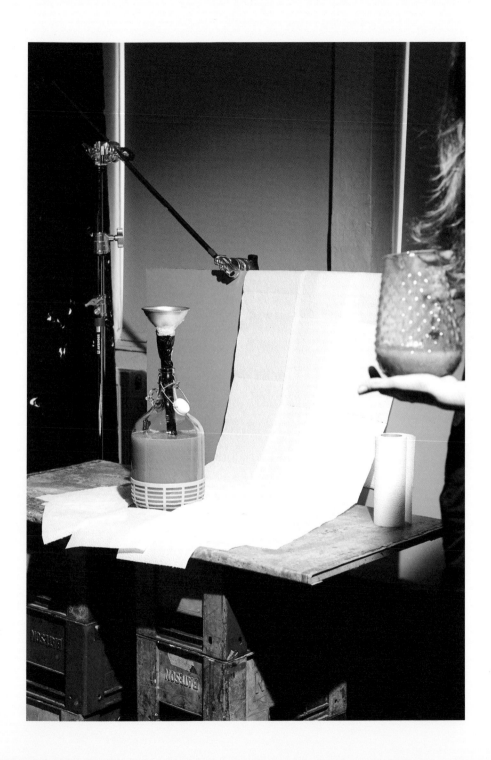

AILMENT INDEX

DEHYDRATION/THIRST

Probiotic Coffee *71*
Hydration Tonic *82*
Homemade Alka Seltzer *5*
Salvation Shrubs *6*
Mexican Medicine*93*
After Dinner Tonic *101*
Make Your Own Probiotics *117*
Fever Grass Tonic *125*
Spicy Thai Tonic *135*

FLUID RETENTION

Turmeric Tamarind Tonic *44*
Hydration Tonic *82*
Homemade Alka Seltzer *85*
Salvation Shrubs *86*
Detox Tonic *98*
Tummy Tonic *102*
Night Nurse *130*
Winter Tea *140*

EMOTIONAL DISTRESS

Love Potion *48*
Happy Tonic *51*
Arroz Con Leche *52*
Sleepy Tonic *55*
Chill Out Tonic *56*
Rooibos Cinnamon Tonic *62*
Z&T *65*
Chai Turmeric Tonic *72*
Herbal Turmeric Tonic *73*
Turmeric Pepper Milk *143*

FATIGUE

Love Potion *48*
Happy Tonic *51*
Sleepy Tonic *55*
Arroz Con Leche *52*
Rooibos Cinnamon Tonic *62*
Z&T *65*
Make Your Own Cold Brew *66*
Probiotic Coffee *71*
Chai Turmeric Tonic *72*
Herbal Turmeric Tonic *73*
Night Nurse *130*

HOT WEATHER

Make Your Own Cold Brew *66*
Probiotic Coffee *71*
Hydration Tonic *82*
Salvation Shrubs *86*
Mexican Medicine *93*
After Dinner Tonic *101*
Tummy Tonic *102*
Turmeric Cream Soda *109*
Overeater's Tonic *115*
Fever Grass Tonic *125*
Spicy Thai Tonic *135*

HEADACHES

Rooibos Cinnamon Tonic *62*
Herbal Turmeric Tonic *73*
Fever Grass Tonic *125*
Night Nurse *130*
Grandma's Tonic *134*

INDIGESTION/UPSET STOMACHS/NAUSEA/DIARRHOEA

Homemade Alka Seltzer *85*
Salvation Shrubs *86*
Mexican Medicine *93*
After Dinner Tonic *101*
Tummy Tonic *102*
Turmeric Cream Soda *109*
Digestive Bitters *101*
Overeater's Tonic *115*
Make Your Own Probiotics *117*
Fermented Honey *144*

WEIGHT LOSS

Turmeric Tamarind Tonic *41*
Rooibos Cinnamon Tonic *62*
Z&T *65*
Hydration Tonic *82*
Salvation Shrubs *86*
Liver Tonic *90*
Detox Tonic *98*
After Dinner Tonic *101*
Digestive Bitters *101*
Overeater's Tonic *115*
Fever Grass Tonic *125*
Make Your Own Probiotics *117*
Prevention Tonic *126*
Grandma's Tonic *134*
Spicy Thai Tonic *135*
Turmeric Pepper Milk *143*

MAIN INDEX

THANK YOU, THANK YOU

To anybody that's ever relished a bottle of Turmeric Tamarind Tonic.

To Dan Buckley, my friend and mentor, for everything. I am forever grateful and look forward to many more endeavours (and beers).

To the dream team behind this book: Dan Buckley (Thumbcrumble), Patricia Niven, James Le Beau-Morley, Olivia Bennett , Jessica Griffiths, Jacqui Melville, and Kajal Mistry for making it happen.

To Nick and Camilla Barnard, for always encouraging me to take my passion to new heights, and the continuous support and mentorship. You are an inspiration.

To Mum and Dad, for your juxtaposing views on what constitutes health, and for keeping my feet firmly on the ground.

To my very first stockist and friend Alex Hely-Hutchinson, for setting the girl-boss bar so high, and for your continuous advice and encouragement.

To my close friends and family, for your patience with the rollercoaster of emotions that is starting up your own business, and writing this book, as well as for your unique views and inputs.

To Annabel Green, for letting me brew over 100 batches of tonic in your kitchen! To Bertel Haugen and Luke Suddards for your imparted wisdom and recipes. And to Tanya Dib, for being there most steps of the way.